Clinical Practice Guidelines in Mental Health

A guide to their use in improving care

Edited by

Paula Whitty

Senior Lecturer in Epidemiology and Public Health
Centre for Health Services Research
University of Newcastle upon Tyne

and

Martin Eccles

William Leech Professor of Primary Care Research
Centre for Health Services Research
University of Newcastle upon Tyne

Forewords by

Professor Sir Michael Rawlins
and
Professor Louis Appleby

Radcliffe Publishing

Oxford • San Francisco

Radcliffe Publishing Ltd
18 Marcham Road
Abingdon
Oxon OX14 1AA
United Kingdom

www.radcliffe-oxford.com
Electronic catalogue and worldwide online ordering.

British Library Cataloguing in Publication Data

A catalogue record for this book is available from the British Library.

ISBN 1 85775 837 4

Typeset by Anne Joshua & Associates, Oxford
Printed and bound by TJ International Ltd, Padstow, Cornwall

Contents

Foreword

I have made no secret of my belief that the real impact of the National Institute for Clinical Excellence (NICE) will be through its clinical practice guidelines. If we can eventually develop a whole suite of National Health Service (NHS) guidelines covering all the major areas of morbidity and mortality, and provided they are fully implemented in routine clinical care, NICE will have made a real difference.

My vision, though, will not be easy to realise. Despite the progress that has been made over the past few years, the methodology for clinical practice guideline development requires further investigation. This particularly applies to economic evaluation where there is much to be done in developing both the theoretical basis, and the practical application. Moreover, experience in guideline development, generally, is currently limited to small numbers of experts and enthusiasts. As a consequence, even if unlimited resources were available, it would be impossible for the UK's NHS to mount a guideline development covering 'all the major areas of morbidity and mortality'. And, despite considerable effort, we do not really know how to ensure that clinical practice guidelines can best be implemented into routine patient care.

The production, by Paula Whitty and Martin Eccles, of *Clinical Practice Guidelines in Mental Health* goes a long way towards realising my ambitions. With over 50 clinical practice guidelines in development, the UK's National Health Service has probably the largest guideline programme of any healthcare system in the world. Although seemingly directed towards mental health, this book has universal applicability and will be invaluable to anyone brave (or foolish) enough to get involved with guideline development and implementation.

Professor Sir Michael Rawlins
Chairman
National Institute for Clinical Excellence
March 2004

Foreword

One of the most important policy initiatives of recent years has been the commitment to evidence-based practice. But what do we mean by evidence, how much is enough, and how is it translated into clinical behaviour?

One challenge facing evidence-based practice is that there are inevitably gaps in evidence in some of the areas that are most in need of guidance – for example, where there is no consensus on best practice or a clash between patient opinion and conventional research, or where a clinical problem is suddenly urgent. It is important to get guidance out to the field when it is needed, not only when it is perfect. But new ways of working will not carry the confidence of health professionals if the evidence they are based upon is seen as flimsy or incomplete. Being pragmatic on the one hand and scientifically rigorous on the other is not easy, but that is the task for guideline developers.

Then there is the challenge of changing how clinicians work. Health staff are not automatons and they need more than objective facts if they are to stop doing one thing and start doing another. After all, they have their clinical experiences to draw on and they need to make judgements about what will benefit an individual patient. Putting guidelines into practice, understanding the human factor in applying knowledge, is the skill that the NHS now has to learn.

Paula Whitty and Martin Eccles have produced a guide to guidelines and made it highly readable as well as useful. It covers a wide range of topics including the nuts and bolts of guideline development, potential pitfalls of using or not using guidelines, details of the National Institute for Clinical Excellence and its collaborating centres, reference to equivalent work in Scotland and feedback on the process of using guidelines at trust and primary care level. The authors have achieved something important and useful: their book is accessible to all those who need to read it – managers, clinicians and trainees.

Healthcare is changing fast and all of us who deliver it need help in making sense of mushrooming research and conflicting findings. The great Canadian doctor Sir William Osler once advised clinicians never to be the first or last to use a new treatment. A hundred years later, clinical guidelines have the same aim.

Professor Louis Appleby
National Director for Mental Health
March 2004

About the editors

Dr Paula Whitty
Senior Lecturer in Epidemiology and Public Health
Centre for Health Services Research
School of Population and Health Sciences
University of Newcastle upon Tyne
and Director of Clinical Governance
Newcastle, North Tyneside and Northumberland Mental Health NHS Trust
Email: p.m.whitty@ncl.ac.uk

Professor Martin Eccles
William Leech Professor of Primary Care Research
and Professor of Clinical Effectiveness
Centre for Health Services Research
School of Population and Health Sciences
University of Newcastle upon Tyne
Email: martin.eccles@ncl.ac.uk

About the contributors

Professor Gene Feder
Professor of Primary Care Research and Development
Institute of Community Health Sciences
Barts and The London
Queen Mary's School of Medicine and Dentistry, London
Email: g.s.feder@qmul.ac.uk

Dr Simon Gilbody
Senior Lecturer in Mental Health Services Research
Academic Unit of Psychiatry
University of Leeds, Leeds
Email: s.m.gilbody@leeds.ac.uk

Professor Chris Griffiths
Professor of Primary Care
Department of General Practice and Primary Care
Barts and The London
Queen Mary's School of Medicine and Dentistry, London
Email: c.j.griffiths@qmul.ac.uk

Dr Hugh Griffiths
Former Joint Medical Director
Newcastle, North Tyneside and Northumberland Mental Health NHS Trust
and Director of Policy and Knowledge Management
NHS Clinical Governance Support Team, Leicester
Email: hugh.griffiths@ncgst.nhs.uk

Professor Jeremy Grimshaw
Director of the Clinical Epidemiology Program
at the Ottawa Health Research Institute and of the Center for Best Practices
Institute of Population Health
University of Ottawa
Ottawa, Ontario, Canada
Email: jgrimshaw@ohri.ca

Professor Richard Grol
Center for Quality of Care Research
Universities of Nijmegen and Maastricht
Nijmegen, The Netherlands
Email: r.grol@wok.umcn.nl

Professor Brian S Hurwitz
D'Oyly Carte Professor of Medicine and the Arts
Department of English Language and Literature
King's College London, London
Email: brian.hurwitz@kcl.ac.uk

Professor Allen Hutchinson
Professor of Public Health Medicine
School of Health and Related Research
University of Sheffield, Sheffield
Email: allen.hutchinson@shef.ac.uk

Dr Tim Kendall
Co-Director
National Collaborating Centre for Mental Health
The Royal College of Psychiatrists' Research Unit, London
Email: tim2.kendall@virgin.net

Dr Gillian Leng
Guidelines Programme Director
National Institute for Clinical Excellence (NICE), London
Email: gillian.leng@nice.nhs.uk

Professor Peter Littlejohns
Clinical Director
National Institute for Clinical Excellence (NICE), London
Email: p.littlejohns@nice.nhs.uk

Dr Carole Longson
Appraisals Programme Director
National Institute for Clinical Excellence, London
Email: clongson@nice.nhs.uk

Professor James Mason
Director
National Guideline Research and Development Unit
Centre for Health Services Research
University of Newcastle upon Tyne, Newcastle upon Tyne
Email: james.mason@ncl.ac.uk

Dr Roger Paxton
Director of Psychological Services
and Director of Research and Development
Newcastle, North Tyneside and Northumberland Mental Health NHS Trust
Morpeth
Email: roger.paxton@nmht.nhs.uk

Dr Steve Pilling
Co-Director
National Collaborating Centre for Mental Health
CORE, Sub-Department of Clinical Health Psychology
University College London, London
Email: s.pilling@ucl.ac.uk

Dr Paul G Shekelle
Veterans Affairs Health Services Research & Development Service
West LA VAMC (111G)
Los Angeles, CA, USA
Email: paul_shekelle@rand.org

Joanne Topalian
Programme Manager – Patient Involvement
Scottish Intercollegiate Guidelines Network (SIGN)
Edinburgh
Email: j.topalian@sign.ac.uk

Dr Sara Twaddle
Director
Scottish Intercollegiate Guidelines Network (SIGN)
Edinburgh
Email: s.twaddle@sign.ac.uk

Professor Andre Tylee
Professor of Primary Care Mental Health
Health Services Research Department
Institute of Psychiatry
London
Email: a.tylee@iop.kcl.ac.uk

Dr Paul Walters
MRC Clinical Research Training Fellow
Health Services Research Department
Institute of Psychiatry
London
Email: p.walters@iop.kcl.ac.uk

Professor Steven H Woolf
Departments of Family Practice, Preventive Medicine and Community Health
Virginia Commonwealth University
Richmond, VA, USA
Email: swoolf@vcu.edu

Acknowledgement

Jeremy Grimshaw holds a Canada Research Chair in Health Knowledge Transfer and Uptake.

Introduction

Paula Whitty
Martin Eccles

Over the last 10 years, clinical practice guidelines have increasingly become a familiar part of healthcare. Every day, clinical decisions at the bedside, rules of operation at hospitals and clinics, and health spending by governments and insurers are being influenced by guidelines. As defined by the USA Institute of Medicine, clinical practice guidelines are 'systematically developed statements to assist practitioner and patient decisions about appropriate healthcare for specific clinical circumstances'.[1] They may offer concise instructions on which diagnostic or screening tests to order, how to provide medical or surgical services, how long to hospitalise patients, or other details of clinical practice. Mental healthcare is no exception: one of the earliest 'evidence-based' guidelines produced in the US was on depression[2] and the England and Wales National Institute for Clinical Excellence's (NICE) portfolio of guidelines in mental health is now beginning to accumulate.

As guidelines diffuse into medicine, there are important lessons to learn from the first-hand experience of those who develop, evaluate and use them.[3] This book aims to reflect on these lessons. The broad interest in clinical practice guidelines has its origin in issues that most healthcare systems face: rising healthcare costs, fuelled by increased demand for care, more expensive technologies, and an ageing population; variations in service delivery among providers, hospitals and geographic regions, and the presumption that at least some of this variation stems from inappropriate care, either over- or under-use of services; and the intrinsic desire of healthcare professionals to offer, and patients to receive, the best care possible. Clinicians, policy makers and commissioners see guidelines as a tool for making care more consistent and efficient and for closing the gap between what clinicians do and what scientific evidence supports. The potential benefits and harms of clinical practice guidelines are considered in Chapter 1.

Discerning users of clinical practice guidelines scrutinise the methods by which they are developed.[4,5] Guideline development groups that do not follow a systematic methodology tend to recommend what a consensus of experts *believe* is good for patients, not necessarily what the evidence supports. Such opinion-based methods, although common, are more vulnerable to bias and conflicts of interest than evidence-based methods that link recommendations directly to data.[6,7] Evidence-based methods emphasise explicitness: they document the strength of the evidence (e.g. by assigning codes or other ratings), offer 'balance sheets' to quantify the potential benefits and harms of available options,[8] acknowledge when recommendations are opinion based and clarify gaps in the evidence. The production of evidence-based clinical practice guidelines is expensive and time consuming. However, by their methods they should maximise validity and minimise bias (although this has not been formally tested). Methods of guideline development are discussed in Chapter 2.

The consideration of benefits and harms within guidelines should extend beyond purely clinical considerations. Guidelines do not exist in a cost-free world and always have economic implications. Chapter 3 discusses the treatment of economic considerations within guideline development.

Chapter 4 moves on to consider aspects of clinical practice guidelines that, in discussions about guidelines, are frequently raised as areas of concern – the legal, emotional and political aspects of clinical practice guidelines.

A fundamental problem is whether clinical practice guidelines developed by any means actually change practice behavior. Simply publishing guidelines has a modest, if any, effect on those who read them.[3,9] To be effective instruments for change, clinical practice guidelines must usually be coupled with active implementation strategies that promote provider acceptance (e.g. professional endorsement, educational outreach, local adaptation), provide implementation tools (e.g. written care pathways, wall charts) and enable or reinforce behaviour change (e.g. computerised reminder systems, audit, feedback).[9] Methods of implementing guidelines, a subject too often ignored by those who develop clinical guidelines,[10] are explored in Chapter 5.

Within England and Wales, NICE now has a prominent role in the co-ordination and development of clinical guidance, both as clinical practice guidelines and as technology appraisals. The Institute's guidelines in the field of mental health are developed by the National Collaborating Centre (NCC) for Mental Health. In Scotland national guidelines are developed by the Scottish Intercollegiate Guidelines Network (SIGN). Since 1993 SIGN has built a programme of more than 60 guidelines. The roles and activities of NICE are described in Chapter 6. Chapter 8 covers the approach to guideline development taken by the NCC for Mental Health and also discusses some of the particular challenges in developing clinical guidelines in this area. Chapter 7 describes the approach and activities of SIGN.

The final two chapters cover the issues of using guidelines in the field of mental health within the NHS. There is very little published on the experience of using guidelines in specialist mental health services, so Chapter 9 provides two case studies from the perspective of a specialist mental health trust. The practical implications of implementing the findings, from a recent systematic review of guidelines, educational and organisational interventions to improve the management of depression in primary care[11,12] are described and discussed in Chapter 10.

Whether you are a specialist mental health professional or a primary care professional who deals with mental health issues on a regular basis, this book should be of interest to you. Mental health service users may also find this book helpful. When appropriate, clinical practice guidelines can improve the health of people with mental health problems, as long as they are rigorously developed and energetically implemented. The aim of this book is to help you better understand this process and to provide examples and ideas for how you might use guidelines in your own practice and setting.

References

1 Field MJ and Lohr KN (eds) (1990) *Clinical Practice Guidelines: directions for a new program*. Institute of Medicine, Committee to Advise the Public Health Service on Clinical Practice Guidelines. National Academy Press, Washington, DC.

2 Agency for Health Care Policy and Research. Depression Guideline Panel (1993) *Depression in Primary Care: detection and diagnosis*. Clinical Guideline Number 5. AHCPR Publication No. 93–0550. AHCPR, Rockville, MD.

3 Field MJ and Lohr KN (eds) (1992) *Guidelines for Clinical Practice: from development to use*. Institute of Medicine, Committee on Clinical Practice Guidelines. National Academy Press, Washington, DC.

4 Hayward RSA, Wilson MC, Tunis SR *et al.* (1995) Users' guide to the medical literature. VIII. How to use clinical practice guidelines. A. Are the recommendations valid? *J Am Med Assoc.* **274**: 570–4.

5 Cluzeau FA, Littlejohns P, Grimshaw JM *et al.* (1999) Development and application of a generic methodology to assess the quality of clinical guidelines. *Int J Qual Health Care.* **11**: 21–8.

6 Shaneyfelt TM, Mayo-Smith MF and Rothwangl J (1999) Are guidelines following guidelines? The methodological quality of clinical practice guidelines in the peer-reviewed medical literature. *J Am Med Assoc.* **281**: 1900–5.

7 Grilli R, Magrini N, Penna A *et al.* (2000) Practice guidelines developed by specialty societies: the need for a critical appraisal. *Lancet.* **355**: 103–6.

8 Eddy DM (1990) Comparing benefits and harms: the balance sheet. *J Am Med Assoc.* **263**: 2493, 2498, 2501.

9 Grimshaw JM, Thomas RE, Maclennan G *et al.* (2004) Effectiveness and efficiency of guideline dissemination and implementation strategies. *Health Technol Assess.* **8**(6).

10 Grol R (1997) Beliefs and evidence in changing clinical practice. *BMJ.* **315**: 418–21.

11 NHS Centre for Reviews and Dissemination (2002) Improving the recognition and management of depression in primary care. *Effect Health Care.* **7**(5).

12 Gilbody S, Whitty P, Grimshaw J *et al.* (2003) Educational and organizational interventions to improve the management of depression in primary care: a systematic review. *J Am Med Assoc.* **289**: 3145–51.

Chapter 1

The potential benefits, limitations and harms of clinical practice guidelines

Steven H Woolf, Martin Eccles, Richard Grol, Allen Hutchinson and Jeremy Grimshaw

The unbridled enthusiasm for guidelines, and the unrealistic expectations about what they will accomplish, frequently betray inexperience and unfamiliarity with their limitations and potential hazards. Naïve consumers of guidelines accept official recommendations at face value, especially when they carry the imprimatur of prominent professional groups or government bodies. However, a growing awareness of their limitations and harms has done little to stem the rapid promulgation of guidelines around the world. It is therefore appropriate to begin a book on clinical practice guidelines by considering their potential benefits and harms.

Potential benefits of clinical practice guidelines

The principal benefit of guidelines is to improve the quality of care received by patients. Whilst it is clear that in the context of rigorous evaluations clinical practice guidelines can improve the quality of patient care,[1,2] whether they achieve this in daily practice is less clear. This is partly because patients, doctors, commissioners and managers define quality differently and because current evidence about the effectiveness of guidelines is incomplete.

Potential benefits for patients

For patients (and nearly everyone else in healthcare), the greatest benefit that could be achieved by guidelines is to improve health outcomes. Guidelines that promote interventions of proven benefit and discourage ineffective ones have the potential to decrease morbidity and premature mortality, and improve quality of life, at least for some conditions. Guidelines can also improve the consistency of care; studies around the world show that the frequency with which procedures are performed varies dramatically among doctors, specialties and geographical regions, even after controlling for case mix.[3] Patients with identical clinical problems receive different care depending on their clinician, hospital or locale. Guidelines offer a remedy, making it more likely that patients will be cared for in the same manner regardless of where or by whom they are treated.

Clinical practice guidelines offer patients other benefits. Those accompanied by 'consumer' versions (lay language leaflets, audiotapes or videos), or publicised in magazines, news reports and Internet sites, inform patients and the public about what their clinicians should be doing. Increasingly lay guidelines summarise the benefits and harms of available options, along with estimates of the probability or magnitude of potential outcomes.[4] Such guidelines empower patients to make more informed healthcare choices and to consider their personal needs and preferences in selecting the best option. Indeed, clinicians may first learn about new guidelines (or be reminded of oversights) when patients enquire about recommendations or treatment options.

Finally, clinical practice guidelines can help patients by influencing public policy. Guidelines call attention to under-recognised health problems, clinical services and preventive interventions, and to neglected patient populations and high-risk groups. Services that were not previously offered to patients may be made available as a response to newly released guidelines. Clinical practice guidelines developed with attention to the public good can promote distributive justice, advocating better delivery of services to those in need. In a cash-limited healthcare system, guidelines that improve the efficiency of healthcare free up resources needed for other (more equitably distributed) healthcare services.

Potential benefits for healthcare professionals

Clinical practice guidelines can improve the quality of clinical decisions. They offer explicit recommendations for clinicians who are uncertain about how to proceed, overturn the beliefs of doctors accustomed to outdated practices, improve the consistency of care and provide authoritative recommendations that reassure practitioners about the appropriateness of their treatment policies. Guidelines based on a critical appraisal of scientific evidence (evidence-based guidelines) clarify which interventions are of proven benefit and document the quality of the supporting data. They alert clinicians to interventions unsupported by good science, reinforce the importance and methods of critical appraisal and call attention to ineffective, dangerous and wasteful practices.

Clinical practice guidelines can support quality improvement activities. The first step in designing quality assessment tools (e.g. audits, care pathways, standing orders) is to reach agreement on how patients should be treated, often by developing a guideline. Guidelines are a common point of reference for prospective and retrospective audits of clinician or hospital practices: the tests, therapies and treatment goals recommended in guidelines provide ready process measures (review criteria) for rating compliance with best care practices.[5]

Medical researchers benefit from the spotlight that evidence-based guidelines shine on gaps in the evidence. The methods of guideline development that feature systematic reviews focus attention on key research questions that must be answered to establish the effectiveness of an intervention[6] and highlight gaps in the identified literature. Critical appraisal of the evidence identifies design flaws in existing studies. Identifying the presence and absence of evidence can redirect the work of investigators and encourage funding agencies to support studies that fulfil this effectiveness-based agenda.

Finally, there are some uses of clinical practice guidelines that straddle the boundary between benefits and harms. Clinicians may seek secular (and even self-serving) benefits from guidelines. In some healthcare systems, guidelines prompt government or private payers to provide coverage or physician reimbursement for services. Specialties engaged in 'turf' wars to gain ownership over specific procedures or treatments may publish a guideline to affirm their role. Clinicians may turn to guidelines for medicolegal protection or to reinforce their position in dealing with administrators who disagree with their practice policies.

Potential benefits for healthcare systems

Healthcare systems that provide services, and government bodies and private insurers that pay for them, have found clinical guidelines potentially effective in improving efficiency (often by standardising care) and optimising value for money.[7] Implementation of certain guidelines reduces outlays for hospitalisation, prescription drugs, surgery and other procedures. Publicising adherence to guidelines may also improve public image, sending messages of commitment to excellence and quality. Such messages can promote goodwill, political support and (in some healthcare systems) revenue. Many believe that the economic motive behind clinical practice guidelines is the principal reason for their popularity.

Potential limitations and harms of guidelines

The most important limitation of guidelines is that the recommendations may be wrong (or at least wrong for individual patients). Setting aside human considerations, such as inadvertent oversights by busy or weary guideline group members, guideline developers may err in determining what is best for patients for three important reasons.

First, scientific evidence about what to recommend is often lacking, misleading or misinterpreted. Only a small subset of what is done in healthcare has been tested in appropriate, well-designed studies. Where studies do exist, the findings may be misleading because of design flaws that contribute to bias or poor generalisability. Guideline development groups often lack the time, resources and skills to gather and scrutinise every last piece of evidence. Even when the data are certain, recommendations for or against interventions will involve subjective value judgements when weighing the benefits against the harms. The value judgement made by a guideline development group may be the wrong choice for individual patients.

Second, recommendations are influenced by the opinions and clinical experience and composition of the guideline development group. Tests and treatments that experts *believe* are good for patients may in practice be inferior to other options, ineffective or even harmful. The beliefs to which experts ascribe, often in the face of conflicting data, can fall victim to misconceptions and personal recollections that misrepresent population norms.[8]

Third, patients' needs may not be the only priority in making recommendations. Practices that are suboptimal from the patient's perspective may be recommended to help control costs, serve societal needs or protect special interests (e.g. physicians, risk managers, politicians).

The promotion of flawed guidelines by practitioners, commissioners, private payers or healthcare systems can encourage, if not institutionalise, the delivery of ineffective, harmful or wasteful interventions. The same parties that stand to benefit from guidelines (patients, healthcare professionals, the healthcare system) may all be harmed.

Potential harms to patients

Patients are most endangered by flawed clinical practice guidelines. Recommendations that do not take due account of the evidence can result in suboptimal, ineffective or harmful practices which, if followed, deny patients their best care. Inflexible guidelines can harm by leaving insufficient room for clinicians to tailor care to patients' personal circumstances and medical or psychiatric history. What is best for patients overall, as recommended in guidelines, may be inappropriate for individuals; blanket recommendations, rather than a menu of options or recommendations for shared decision making, ignore patient preferences.[9] Thus the frequently touted benefit of clinical guidelines – more consistent practice patterns and reduced variation – may come at the expense of reducing individualised care for patients with special needs. Lay versions of guidelines, if improperly constructed and worded, may mislead or confuse patients and disrupt the clinician–patient relationship.

Clinical practice guidelines can adversely affect public policy for patients. Recommendations against an intervention may lead providers to drop access to, or coverage for, services. Imprudent recommendations for costly interventions may displace limited resources needed for other services of greater value to patients. The tendency for guidelines to focus attention on specific health issues is subject to misuse by proponents and advocacy groups, giving the public (and health professionals) the wrong impression about the relative importance of diseases and effectiveness of interventions.

Potential harms to healthcare professionals

Flawed clinical practice guidelines harm practitioners by providing inaccurate scientific information and clinical advice, thereby compromising the quality of care. They may encourage ineffective, harmful or wasteful interventions. Even when guidelines are correct, clinicians often find them inconvenient and time-consuming to use. Conflicting guidelines from different professional bodies can also confuse and frustrate practitioners.[10] Outdated recommendations may perpetuate outmoded practices and technologies.

Clinical practice guidelines can also hurt clinicians professionally. Auditors and managers may unfairly judge the quality of care based on criteria from invalid guidelines. The well-intentioned effort to make guidelines explicit and practical encourages the injudicious use of certain words (e.g. 'should' versus 'may'), arbitrary numbers (e.g. months of treatment, interval between screening tests), and simplistic algorithms when supporting evidence may be lacking. Algorithms that reduce patient care into a sequence of binary ('yes/no') decisions often do injustice to the complexity of healthcare and the parallel and iterative thought processes inherent in clinical judgement. Words, numbers and simplistic algorithms can be used by those who judge clinicians to repudiate unfairly those who, for legitimate reasons, follow different practice policies.

Guidelines carry economic implications. Referral guidelines can shift patients from one specialty to another. A negative (or neutral) recommendation may prompt providers to withdraw availability or coverage. A theoretical concern is that clinicians may be sued for not adhering to guidelines although, as discussed in Chapter 4 of this book, this has not yet become a reality.

Guidelines can harm medical investigators and scientific progress if further research is inappropriately discouraged. Guidelines that conclude that a procedure or treatment lacks evidence of benefit may be misinterpreted by funding bodies as grounds for not investing in further research and for not supporting efforts to refine previously ineffective technologies.

Potential harms to healthcare systems

Healthcare systems, commissioners and private payers may be harmed by guidelines if following them escalates utilisation, compromises operating efficiency and/or wastes limited resources. Some clinical practice guidelines, especially those developed by medical and other groups unconcerned about financing, may advocate costly interventions that are unaffordable or that cut into resources needed for more effective services.

Conclusions

In the face of these mixed consequences, attitudes about whether clinical practice guidelines are good or bad for healthcare vary from one group to another. Guidelines produced by government or payers to control spiralling costs may constitute responsible public policy but may be resented by clinicians and patients as an invasion of personal autonomy. Guidelines developed by specialists may seem self-serving, biased and threatening to generalists. To specialists, guidelines developed without their input suffer from inadequate content expertise. Inflexible guidelines with rigid rules about what is appropriate are popular with some managers, quality auditors and lawyers but are described as 'cookbook medicine' by clinicians faced with non-uniform clinical problems and as invalid by those who cite the lack of supporting data.

Clinical practice guidelines are only one option for improving the quality of care. Too often, advocates view guidelines as a 'magic bullet' for healthcare problems and ignore more effective solutions. Clinical practice guidelines make sense when practitioners are unclear about appropriate practice and when scientific evidence can provide an answer. They are a poor remedy in other settings.

References

1 Effective Health Care (1994) *Implementing Clinical Practice Guidelines*. Bulletin No 8. University of Leeds, Leeds.
2 Grimshaw JM, Thomas RE, Maclennan G *et al.* (2004) Effectiveness and efficiency of guideline dissemination and implementation strategies. *Health Technol Assess*. 8(6).
3 Chassin MR, Brook RH, Park RE *et al.* (1986) Variations in the use of medical and surgical services by the Medicare population. *N Engl J Med.* 314: 285–90.
4 Entwistle VA, Watt IS, Davis H *et al.* (1998) Developing information materials to present the findings of technology assessments to consumers: the experience of the NHS Centre for Reviews and Dissemination. *Int J Tech Assess Health Care.* 14: 47–70.
5 Agency for Health Care Policy and Research (1995) *Using Clinical Practice Guidelines to Evaluate Quality of Care. Volume 1: Issues.* US Department of Health and Human Services, Public Health Services, Rockville, MD.
6 Cook DJ, Mulrow CD and Haynes RB (1997) Systematic reviews: synthesis of best evidence for clinical practice. *Ann Intern Med.* 126: 376–80.
7 Shapiro DW, Lasker RD, Bindman AB *et al.* (1993) Containing costs while improving quality of care: the role of profiling and practice guidelines. *Ann Rev Public Health.* 14: 219–41.

8   Kane RL (1995) Creating practice guidelines: the dangers of over-reliance on expert judgment. *J Law Med Ethics*. **23**: 62–4.

9   Woolf SH (1997) Shared decision-making: the case for letting patients decide which choice is best. *J Fam Pract*. **45**: 205–8.

10 Feder G (1994) Management of mild hypertension: which guidelines to follow? *BMJ*. **308**: 470–1.

Chapter 2

Developing guidelines

Paul G Shekelle, Martin Eccles, Steven H Woolf and
Jeremy Grimshaw

The rationale for developing guidelines is to achieve better health outcomes for patients or greater value for money than would have been
achieved in the absence of guidelines. Therefore the methods of guideline
development should ensure that treating patients according to the guidelines will achieve the outcomes that are desired. Three important issues
underpin the development of valid and useable guidelines.

1   The development of guidelines requires sufficient resources in the form
    of both persons with a wide range of skills, including expert clinicians,
    health services researchers and group process leaders, and financial
    resources.
2   A systematic review of the evidence should be at the heart of every
    guideline.
3   The expert group assembled to translate the evidence into a guideline
    should be multidisciplinary.

There are five steps in the initial development of an evidence-based
guideline (Box 2.1). A guideline will also require review after an appropriate period of time. The dissemination, implementation and evaluation
of practice guidelines will be discussed in Chapter 5.

Box 2.1: Five steps in clinical practice guideline development

- Identifying and refining the subject area of a guideline
- Convening and running guideline development groups
- Assessing the evidence about the clinical question or condition
- Translating the evidence into a clinical practice guideline
- External review of the guideline

Identifying and refining the subject area of a guideline

Prioritising topics for guideline development

Guidelines can be developed for a wide range of subjects. Clinical areas can be concerned with conditions (depression, diabetes, coronary artery disease) or procedures (electroconvulsive therapy, hysterectomy, coronary artery bypass surgery). Given the large number of potential areas, some form of prioritisation is needed to select a particular area for guideline development. Potential areas for clinical practice guideline development can emerge from an assessment of the major causes of morbidity and mortality for a given population, uncertainty about the appropriateness of healthcare processes or the evidence that they are effective in improving patient outcomes, or the need to conserve resources in providing care.

Refining the subject area of a guideline

However, once the topic for guideline development is identified, it will usually need to be refined before beginning an assessment of the evidence in order to answer exact questions. This can be achieved in a number of ways. The usual way is by a dialogue among clinicians, patients and the potential end-users or evaluators of the guideline. Discussions about the scope of the guideline will also take place within the guideline development panel.

Failure to carry out this refinement runs the risk of leaving the clinical condition or question too broad in scope. For example, a guideline on 'the management of diabetes' could conceivably cover both primary, secondary and tertiary care elements of management and multiple aspects of management, such as screening, diagnosis, dietary management, drug therapy, risk factor management or indications for referral to a consultant. While all of these could be legitimate areas for guideline development, such a task would be considerable; therefore a group needs to be clear which areas are and are not within the scope of its activities. It is possible to develop guidelines that are both broad in scope and evidence based, but to do so usually requires a considerable investment in both time and money, both of which are frequently underestimated by inexperienced developers of evidence-based clinical practice guidelines.

One method to both define the clinical question of interest and identify exactly for which processes evidence needs to be collected and assessed is the construction of models or causal pathways.[1] A causal pathway is a diagram that illustrates the linkages between intervention(s) of interest and the intermediate, surrogate and health outcomes that the interventions are thought to influence. In designing the pathway, guideline developers make explicit the premises on which their assumptions of effectiveness are based and the outcomes (benefits and harms) that they consider important. This identifies the specific questions that must be answered by the evidence to justify conclusions of effectiveness and highlights gaps in the evidence for which future research is needed.

Convening and running guideline development groups

Setting up a guideline development project

To succeed in the task of guideline development it may be necessary to convene more than one group. Potential groups would be a project or management team to undertake the day-to-day running of the work, such as the identification, synthesis and interpretation of relevant evidence, the convening and running of the guideline development groups and the production of the resulting guidelines. Additional guideline development group(s) would undertake the task of producing the guidelines' recommendations in the light of the evidence or its absence. While there is no single right way to set up such groups it is important to ensure that guideline development is adequately resourced, particularly as groups often report underestimating the resources required for the task – both in terms of finance and project management and in terms of general administrative support.

The guideline development group: membership and roles

The composition of a guideline development group can be considered in two ways: by the disciplines of the group members who would be stakeholders in the area of the guideline and by the roles required within the group.

Group members
Identifying stakeholders involves identifying all the groups whose activities would be covered by the guideline or who have other legitimate reasons for having an input into the process. This is important to ensure adequate discussion of the evidence (or its absence) when developing the recommendations in the guideline. There is good evidence that, when presented with the same evidence, a single-specialty group will reach different conclusions than a multidisciplinary group, with the former being systematically biased in favour of performing procedures in which the specialty has a vested interest.[2,3] For example, the conclusions of a group of vascular surgeons favoured the use of carotid endarterectomy more than those of a mixed group of surgeons and medical specialists.[4] There are good theoretical reasons to believe that individuals' biases are better balanced in multidisciplinary groups and that such balance will produce more valid guidelines. Ideally the group should have at least six,

but no more than 12–15, members; too few members limits adequate discussion and too many members makes effective functioning of the group difficult. Under certain circumstances (e.g. when developing guidelines for broad clinical areas) it may be necessary to trade off full representation against the requirement of having a functional group.

Roles

Potential roles required within guideline development groups are: group member, group leader, specialist resource, technical support and administrative support. Group members, as indicated above, are invited to participate as individuals working in their field. Their role is to develop recommendations for practice based upon the available evidence and their knowledge of the practicalities of clinical practice.

The role of the group leader is both to ensure that the group functions effectively (the group process) and that it achieves its aims (the group task). Although guideline groups are often chaired by pre-eminent experts in the topic area, we believe the process is best moderated by someone familiar with (though not necessarily an expert in) the management of the clinical condition and the scientific literature but someone who is not an advocate. Such an individual acts to stimulate discussion and allows the group to identify where true agreement exists, but does not inject their own opinion in the process. This requires someone with both clinical skills and group process skills. There is also evidence that conducting the group meetings using formal group processes rather than informal ones produces different and possibly better outcomes.[5-7]

Guideline processes will require a variety of specialist support at various times and this may be fulfilled by more than one individual. Some of the potential skills required are shown in Box 2.2. Finally, groups will require administrative support for such tasks as preparing papers for meetings, taking notes and arranging venues.

Box 2.2: Skills needed in guideline development

- Literature searching and retrieval
- Epidemiology
- Biostatistics
- Health services research
- Clinical expertise
- Group process expertise
- Writing and editing

Identifying and assessing the evidence

Identifying and assessing the evidence is best done by performing a systematic review. The purpose of a systematic review is to collect all available evidence, assess its potential applicability to the clinical question under consideration, inspect the evidence for susceptibility to bias and extract and summarise the findings (Box 2.3).

Box 2.3: Assessing the evidence

- Collect all of the evidence
- Assess the evidence for relevance
- Assess the evidence for susceptibility to bias
- Extract and summarise evidence about benefits, costs and harms

---

What sort of evidence?

The identification of the clinical questions of interest (using clinical pathways) will help set the boundaries for admissible evidence (the types of study design, the year of publication, etc.). For example, questions of the efficacy of interventions usually mean that randomised controlled trials (RCTs) should be sought, while questions of risk usually mean that prospective cohort studies should be sought. Similarly, studies of interventions need be searched only back until their introduction (for example, newer antipsychotic drugs such as clozapine were introduced in the 1990s while haloperidol has been used for over 30 years).

Where to look for evidence?

The first step in gathering the evidence is to see if a suitable, recent systematic review has already been published.[8] The Cochrane Library includes the Cochrane trials register, database of systematic reviews and the database of abstracts of reviews of effectiveness. Relevant Cochrane review groups should also be contacted to see if a review is in progress.

If a current systematic review is not available, a computerised search of MEDLINE and EMBASE is the usual starting point, using search strategies that have been previously shown to be sensitive for detecting the types of studies one is looking for (though these have only been validated for RCTs).[9] For example, RCTs provide the best evidence to answer questions about the effectiveness of treatments whereas prospective cohort studies provide the best evidence for questions about risk. The Cochrane trials register contains references to over 375,000 clinical trials that have been identified through database and hand searching and represents the best initial source of such studies. As such it should be examined early on in any review process. It is helpful to check the references of all the articles identified to see if there are additional relevant articles not identified by the computerised search. Having experts in the field examine the list of articles helps ensure that there are no obvious omissions. Additional search strategies, including searches for articles published in languages other than English,[10–12] computerised searches of specialised databases, hand searching relevant journals and searching for unpublished material, will, in many cases, yield additional studies, but the resources needed for such activities are considerable and may not be feasible. The cost-effectiveness of various search strategies has not been established. It is best to match the scope of the search strategy to the available resources.

Assessing studies for relevance

The studies identified are then assessed for relevance to the clinical questions of interest and their susceptibility to bias. This is usually a two-step process. The initial screen or sift for relevance (often possible by reading the abstract) narrows the set to those needing a more detailed assessment. In both cases, the use of explicit rather than implicit criteria should improve the reliability of the process. There is some limited empirical evidence that the use of two persons working independently improves the accuracy of this step in data collection.[13]

Susceptibility to bias is dependent upon study design. Randomised controlled trials are by design less susceptible to bias than case series studies for answering questions about the efficacy of interventions.[14,15] Prospective cohort studies are less susceptible to bias than retrospective cohort studies for answering questions about risk. Susceptibility to bias is also affected by the subsequent conduct of a study (e.g. studies in which randomisation is inadequately concealed are more susceptible to bias).[16] Whilst there are many different scoring systems for assessing the quality of studies, there is little empirical evidence about their validity.[17–19] Guideline developers should focus on methodological criteria for which there is empirical evidence of importance.

Summarising evidence

In the last step, data are extracted from the relevant studies on the benefits, harms and, where applicable, costs of the interventions being considered. These are usually presented in a form which facilitates easy comparison of the designs and results of studies. Where appropriate, meta-analysis can be used to summarise results of multiple studies.

Categorising evidence

Summarised evidence is categorised to reflect its underlying susceptibility to bias. This is a shorthand method of conveying to a guideline reader specific aspects of the evidence. A number of such 'strength of evidence' classification schemes exist but empirical supporting evidence only exists for those categorising effectiveness studies.[14,15] Different schemes applied to the same evidence can lead to vastly different conclusions.[20] We suggest that guideline developers should use a limited number of explicit criteria, incorporating those for which there is explicit evidence.

Translating evidence into a clinical practice guideline

Evidence alone is not sufficient to form a recommendation; the evidence needs to be interpreted. Box 2.4 lists the factors that contribute to deriving recommendations within a clinical practice guideline. Since conclusive evidence exists for few healthcare procedures, deriving recommendations solely in areas of strong evidence would lead to a guideline of limited scope or applicability.[21] In certain limited circumstances, this could be sufficient if, for example, the guideline is to recommend the most strongly supported treatments for a given illness. More commonly the evidence needs to be interpreted into a clinical, public health, policy or commissioning context. Therefore, within the guideline development process a decision should be taken about how opinion will be both used and gathered.

Box 2.4: Factors contributing to the process of deriving recommendations

- The nature of the evidence (e.g. its susceptibility to bias)
- The applicability of the evidence to the population of interest (its generalisability)
- Costs
- Knowledge of the healthcare system
- Beliefs and values of the panel

Using and gathering opinion

Opinion will be used both to interpret evidence and to derive recommendations in the absence of evidence. When interpreting evidence, opinion is needed to assess issues such as the generalisability of evidence. For example, opinion is needed to judge to what degree evidence from studies, such as small randomised clinical trials or controlled observational studies, may be generalised or to extrapolate results from a study in one population to the population of interest in the guideline (for example, from a study in a tertiary, academic medical centre population to the community population of interest to potential users of the guideline).

Recommendations based solely on clinical judgement and experience are likely to be more susceptible to bias and self-interest. Therefore, after deciding what role expert opinion is to play, the next step is deciding how to collect and assess expert opinion. Unfortunately, less is known about how to assemble opinion sources than about how to collect and assess published literature and there is no current gold standard method. Best practice is to make the process at least as explicit as possible.

Resource implications and feasibility

In addition to scientific evidence and the opinions of expert clinicians, clinical practice guidelines must often take account of the resource implications and feasibility of interventions. Judgements about whether the costs of tests or treatments are reasonable depend on how cost-effectiveness is defined and calculated, on the perspective taken (e.g. clinicians often view cost implications differently than would payers or society at large) and on the resource constraints of the healthcare system (e.g. cash-limited public versus private insurance-based systems). Feasibility issues worthy of consideration include the time, skills, personnel and equipment necessary for the provider to carry out the recommendations and the ability of patients and systems of care to implement them.

Grading recommendations

It is common to grade each guideline recommendation. Such information provides the user with an indication of the guideline development group's confidence that following the guideline will produce the desired health outcome. While a number of 'strength of recommendation' classification schemes exist, from simple to complex, no classification scheme has been shown to be superior. However, given the factors that contribute to a recommendation (Box 2.4), strong evidence does not always produce a strong recommendation and the classification should allow for this. The classification is probably best done by the group panel using a democratic voting process after group discussion of the strength of the evidence.

External review of the guideline

Prior to finalising the guideline, we believe it important to have external review of the guideline for content validity, clarity and applicability. External reviewers should cover three areas.

1 Persons with clinical content expertise, who can review the guideline to verify the completeness of the literature review and to ensure clinical sensibility.

2   Persons expert in systematic reviews and/or guideline development, who can review the method by which the guideline was developed.
3   Potential users of the guideline, who can judge the usefulness of the guideline.

Updating of a guideline

This chapter has concentrated on the initial development of an evidence-based guideline. However, with time new evidence will be published and should be incorporated into an updated version of the guideline.[22] There are two potential ways of doing this. Either the guideline can be updated as soon as each and every piece of relevant new evidence is published or a review date is specified in advance as the point at which the systematic review underpinning the guideline is updated. There is empirical evidence that, on average, guidelines go out of date in three to five years.[23] Experience with updating evidence-based guidelines is limited. While the methods may be the same as in the initial development of the guideline, and the resources required may be of a similar magnitude, a recent publication supports using a less expensive mail-only process to solicit expert opinion for updating existing criteria.[24]

Conclusions

We have presented here a combination of the literature about guideline development and the results of our combined experience in guideline development in North America and Britain. The process of guideline development is dynamic and it is likely that ongoing work on both sides of the Atlantic will expand the empirical evidence upon which our decisions about guideline development are based. New advances in understanding the science of systematic reviews, the workings of groups of experts and the relationship between guideline development and implementation are all likely within the next three to five years. We believe, however, that three principles will remain fundamental to the development of valid and useable guidelines.

1   The development of guidelines requires sufficient resources in terms of persons with a wide range of skills, including expert clinicians, health services researchers and group process leaders, and financial support.
2   A systematic review of the evidence should be at the heart of every guideline.
3   The expert group assembled to translate the evidence into a guideline should be multidisciplinary.

References

1 Woolf SH (1994) An organized analytic framework for practice guideline development: using the analytic logic as a guide for reviewing evidence, developing recommendations, and explaining the rationale. In: KA McCormick, SR Moore and RA Siegel (eds) *Methodology Perspectives*, AHCPR Publication No. 95-0009. US Department of Health and Human Services, Agency for Health Care Policy and Research, Washington, DC, pp. 105–13.

2 Kahan JP, Park RE, Leape LL *et al.* (1996) Variations by specialty in physician ratings of the appropriateness and necessity of indications for procedures. *Med Care.* **34**(6): 512–23.

3 Coulter I, Adams A and Shekelle P (1995) Impact of varying panel membership on ratings of appropriateness in consensus panels – a comparison of a multi- and single disciplinary panel. *Health Serv Res.* **30**(4): 577–91.

4 Leape LL, Park RE, Kahan JP *et al.* (1992) Group judgments of appropriateness: the effect of panel composition. *Quality Assur Health Care.* **4**(2): 151–9.

5 Kosecoff JH, Kanouse DE, Rogers WH *et al.* (1987) Effects of the National Institutes of Health Consensus Development Program on physician practice. *J Am Med Assoc.* **258**(19): 2708–13.

6 Shekelle PG and Schriger DL (1996) Evaluating the use of the appropriateness method in the Agency for Health Care Policy and Research clinical practice guideline development process. *Health Serv Res.* **31**(4): 453–68.

7 Shekelle PG, Kravitz RL, Beart J *et al.* (2000) Are nonspecific practice guidelines potentially harmful? A randomised comparison of the effect of nonspecific versus specific guidelines on physician decision making. *Health Serv Res.* **34**(7): 1429–48.

8 Eccles M, Freemantle N and Mason J (2001) Using systematic reviews in clinical guideline development. In: M Egger, G Davey Smith and DG Altman (eds) *Systematic Reviews in Healthcare: meta-analysis in context.* BMJ Books, London.

9 Cochrane Reviewer's Handbook (2003) In: *The Cochrane Library* (database on disk and CD-ROM), The Cochrane Collaboration. Update Software, Oxford.

10 Dickersin K, Scherer R and Lefebvre C (1994) Identifying relevant studies for systematic reviews. *BMJ.* **309**: 1286.

11 Gregoire G, Derderian F and Le Lorier J (1995) Selecting the language of the publications included in a meta-analysis: is there a Tower of Babel bias? *J Clin Epidemiol.* **48**(1): 159–63.

12 Egger M, Zellweger-Zähner, Schneider M *et al.* (1997) Language bias in randomised controlled trials published in English and German. *Lancet.* **350**: 326–9.

13 Strang N, Boissel JP and Uberla K (1997) Inter-reader variation. *5th Annual Cochrane Colloquium Abstract Book.* The Cochrane Collaboration, Oxford, p. 279.

14 Colditz GA, Miller JN and Mosteller F (1989) How study design affects outcomes in comparisons of therapy I: medical. *Stat Med.* **8**: 441–54.

15 Miller JN, Colditz GA and Mosteller F (1989) How study design affects outcomes in comparisons of therapy II: surgical. *Stat Med.* **8**: 455–66.

16 Schulz KF, Chalmers I, Hayes RJ *et al.* (1995) Empirical evidence of bias: dimensions of methodological quality associated with estimates of treatment effects in controlled trials. *J Am Med Assoc.* **273**(5): 408–12.

17 Moher D, Jones A, Cook D *et al.* (1999) Does quality of reports of randomised trials affect estimates of intervention efficacy reported in meta-analyses? *Lancet.* **352**: 609–13.

18 Juni P, Witchi A, Block R *et al.* (1999) The hazards of scoring the quality of clinical trials for meta-analysis. *J Am Med Assoc.* **282**(11): 1054–60.

19 Balk EM, Bonis PA, Moskowitz H *et al.* (2002) Correlation of quality measures with estimates of treatment effect in meta-analyses of randomised controlled trials. *J Am Med Assoc.* **287**(22): 2973–82.

20 Ferreira PH, Ferreira ML, Maher CG *et al.* (2002) Effect of applying different 'levels of evidence' criteria on conclusions of Cochrane reviews of interventions for low back pain. *J Clin Epidemiol.* **55**(11): 1126–9.

21 Shekelle P, Chassin MR and Park RE (1998) Assessing the predictive validity of the RAND/UCLA appropriateness method criteria for performing carotid endarterectomy. *Int J Technol Assess Health Care.* **14**: 707–27.

22 Shekelle P, Eccles MP, Grimshaw JM *et al.* (2001) When should clinical guidelines be updated? *BMJ.* **323**: 155–7.

23 Shekelle PG, Ortiz E, Rhodes S *et al.* (2001) Validity of the Agency for Healthcare Research and Quality clinical practice guidelines: how quickly do guidelines become outdated? *J Am Med Assoc.* **286**(12): 1461–7.

24 Washington DL, Bernstein SJ, Kahan JP *et al.* (2003) Reliability of clinical guideline development using mail-only versus in-person expert panels. *Med Care.* **41**: 1374–81.

Chapter 3

Health economics and clinical practice guidelines

Martin Eccles and James Mason

Unlike other areas of guideline development, there is little practical or theoretical experience to direct the incorporation of cost issues within clinical guidelines. However, the reasons for considering costs are clearly stated by Eddy: 'Health interventions are not free, people are not infinitely rich, and the budgets of (healthcare) programmes are limited. For every dollar's worth of healthcare that is consumed, a dollar will be paid. While these payments can be laundered, disguised or hidden, they will not go away'.[1] Such opportunity costs are not particular to the healthcare system of the USA, but a universal phenomenon; the NHS needs to obtain the best value from finite public funds.

The Committee on Clinical Practice Guidelines[2] recommended that every set of clinical guidelines should include information on the cost implications of the alternative preventive, diagnostic and management strategies for each clinical situation. Its stated rationale was that this information would help potential users to better evaluate the potential consequences of different practices. Although acknowledging that 'The reality is . . . this recommendation poses major methodological and practical challenges', it suggested that, in the process of considering costs, five questions should be examined (Box 3.1).

It then went on to offer a range of reasons as to why guideline developers would have difficulty finding the answers to these questions (Box 3.2).

An additional layer of complexity is then added by acknowledging that the approach to costs and guidelines may vary when developing guidelines for different audiences. Whilst accepting that there will be overlap between groups, typically clinicians and patients will be most interested in cost issues impacting on individual treatment decisions. Whilst this will also be of interest to policy makers, they are likely to have an additional interest in the population cost and health impact of introducing a guideline into a service.

Box 3.1: Issues to be addressed in clinical guidelines

- What evidence suggests that the services are likely to affect outcomes for the condition or intervention being considered?
- Which groups at risk are most likely to experience benefits or harms from the proposed course of care and its side-effects?
- What is known about the effects of different frequencies, duration, dosages or other variations in the intensity of the intervention?
- Which options in the ways services are organised and provided can affect the benefits, harms and costs of services?
- Which benefits, harms and costs can be expected from alternative diagnostic or treatment paths, including watchful waiting or no intervention?

Source: Institute of Medicine (1992)[2]

Box 3.2: Problems confronting guideline developers

- Scientific evidence about benefits and harms is incomplete
- Basic, accurate cost data are scarce for the great majority of clinical conditions and services
- While data on charges may be available, significant analytic steps and assumptions are required to treat charge data as cost data
- Techniques for analysing and projecting costs and cost-effectiveness are complex and only evolving

Source: Institute of Medicine (1992)[2]

Using cost data when developing a clinical practice guideline

Questions about, and limitations of, cost-effectiveness analyses raise the issue of how to use cost data in a guidelines group. Should data be presented alongside recommendations based solely on clinical effectiveness or incorporated into the judgement process of deriving recommendations? Williams[3] and Eddy[1] argue that guidelines based on effectiveness issues and then costed may differ substantially from and be less efficient than guidelines based on cost-effectiveness issues. The complexity of this process, and the reactions it evokes, are reflected by the Committee on Clinical Practice Guidelines' report[2] of 'much debate, and with some vigorous dissent'. There has been no widely accepted successful way of incorporating economic considerations into guidelines.

Clinicians (the key audience) do not appear to think of appropriate healthcare in terms of economic outcomes such as cost-effectiveness ratios. The fact that there is an issue about how healthcare professionals think about, and react to, explicit cost issues in guidelines is understandable. Most healthcare professionals have a limited knowledge of health economics and economic modelling. Guidelines based on clinical effectiveness could be enhanced or undermined by the incorporation of economic considerations, depending on whether they are seen as attempts to achieve cost-effectiveness or cost-containment. It remains a research issue as to how the incorporation of economic considerations will affect the use of guidelines in individual treatment decisions, although the intention is to encourage a more explicit consideration of costs and consequences in each consultation where guidelines are used. British health professionals are not accustomed to this process at anything other than an implicit level, although in recent years cost messages have indirectly impinged more and more through formulary lists or fund-holding initiatives. In the absence of an overarching framework for resource allocation (and in a system where healthcare is provided from general taxation) the first step in moving this process forward is to develop robust methods of incorporating economic issues into clinical practice guidelines.

Building a profile of treatments

The product of the review of evidence, for a guideline development group, should be an appropriate summary or profile of the important consequences of treatment. This may include evidence about clinical outcomes, compliance, quality of life, safety and health service resource use (Box 3.3).

Box 3.3: The profile of treatment attributes addressed in guidelines

- Effectiveness
- Quality of life
- Tolerability
- Safety
- Health service delivery issues (implementation)
- Health service resource use
- Health service costs
- Patient and carer costs

Any aspect of treatment that may be valued by patients or society more broadly should be considered for inclusion in the profile. The list of attributes does not require dogmatic adherence, since different diseases and their treatments will impact upon patient health differently and, pragmatically, data are often unavailable for a number of attributes. However, it is important, early on in the guideline process, to identify the important consequences of alternative strategies of care.

The profile approach leads to simple presentations of cost implications and other consequences that are readily comprehensible to guideline readers of any background. The available evidence on which these presentations are based is not necessarily robust, but by explicitly identifying uncertainties, the presentation of the evidence accurately identifies strengths and weaknesses and end-users of the guideline can easily explore alternative values.

Use of meta-analysis may be possible where the data permit. However, summaries of the evidence may be limited to a narrative-style review where available evidence is poor, uses incompatible assessments of outcome or is inconsistently reported (a qualitative summary). Sometimes the information emerging from the review profile does not provide a clear message and it may be useful to employ some form of modelling to help the guideline development group to explore the implications of treatments more fully.

The review, and need for any subsequent modelling, evolves through group discussion as understanding of the value of treatments emerges.[4] The group uses the profile to explore the incremental costs and consequences of the different healthcare decisions open to them to recommend. Economic analysis is thus used to attempt a robust presentation showing the possible bounds of cost-effectiveness that may result. The range of values used to generate low and high cost-effectiveness estimates reflects the available evidence and the concerns of the guideline development group. Nonetheless, the simplicity of presentation permits simple reworking with different values from the ones used. Recommendations are graded, reflecting the certainty with which the costs and consequences of a medical intervention can be assessed. This practice reflects the desire of group members to have simple, understandable and robust information based on good data.

There may be evidence that health-associated costs borne by patients and carers (e.g. travel and time to receive care, over-the-counter drugs, disability costs) and indirect costs of lost earnings differ significantly between alternative treatments. This should be considered relevant to a treatment decision at least in as much as it may undesirably influence concordance with treatment. There is the possibility that organisational alternatives may shift costs from the health service to individuals and the appropriateness of this may depend on the disease considered and contextual circumstances. Seldom are there adequate data to address costs borne by patients but where this is a concern, these can be described as attributes of treatments.

Profiles and modelling

Traditionally it is the province of health economics to model intermediate and context-specific clinical outcome data, and data from other sources, to explore the overall costs and consequences of treatment alternatives. The measurement of health as an outcome has mushroomed as an academic and clinical pursuit in recent years and has resulted in the development of generic measures that express patient health status (and its changes over time) as a single index (e.g. the quality-adjusted life-year or QALY). Thus, theoretically, health gains could be compared across different diseases and patient groups and cost/QALY estimates could provide a common metric for comparing the value for money of the myriad healthcare interventions available. In principle, it is possible to map clinical data onto generic quality of life scores, model the advancement of disease and produce cost per QALY estimates for each treatment decision. However, a cost/QALY calculation, by seeking to solve a big question (how does one treatment compare with any other treatment for any other disease?), may often be inefficient in terms of the objectives of a guideline. For example, knowing alternative antidepressants are similarly effective, tolerable and safe but have markedly different acquisition costs may be sufficient to make clinically appropriate treatment recommendations.

However, the issue is not a simple 'model/don't model' one. Meta-analysis is a kind of model that makes statistical and clinical assumptions when combining data. A profile of attributes used to help formulate treatment recommendations is one representation of reality. Although the assumptions may be less presumptuous than those found in many decision analyses, an implicit modelling process is being conducted when a guideline development group weighs up the attributes of treatments and formulates recommendations. The difference is one of emphasis: while some health economists may seek to obtain clear, aggregated answers from a complex pattern of information, it is the pattern itself that plays an important part in the clinical decision-making process. Simple modelling exercises may be necessary to enable a guideline development group to interpret the evidence before them. Subsequent readers of the full guideline report should, however, be able to follow and, if they wish, replicate or modify the process.

Reviewing economic analyses

In many fields of healthcare there is a body of economic literature accompanying the clinical studies. As with a review of available clinical trials, it is feasible to have a summary of published economic analyses and methods of assessing and categorising economic studies are being developed. Unlike protocol-driven prospective clinical trials, economic analyses are usually retrospective and the analyst has the choice of how to construct the model and use the data. Qualitatively there is far greater scope for bias, either explicit or implicit, in the process or model construction, reporting of findings and exploration of uncertainty.[5,6] A guideline development process should lead to the best available presentation of the known costs and various physical consequences of treatment alternatives. These data are unlikely to match the baseline assumptions in any published model. Each clinical trial presents unique or independent data and the trials together can be summarised to obtain an overview. Different economic analyses take different cuts at the same clinical data and there is no quantitative way to summarise the findings of all the analyses as the data are not independent. Thus, there is no 'weight of evidence'. Published decision analyses are often not transparent and it can be difficult and time-consuming to validate the findings presented

Assessing the cost impact of a guideline

Policy makers may routinely wish to know the cost impact of implementing a guideline. For example, where a new and expensive treatment is recommended, it might be possible to assess the net cost to the NHS of different levels of uptake of recommendations, alongside the expected benefits. However, the longer term costs and consequences of treatments are often circumspect, making overall cost impact assessments inherently uncertain. Baseline levels of activity may be unknown or locally variable and therefore the level of change resulting from a new guideline becomes largely informed guesswork. Typically clinical practice guidelines will cover the breadth of a clinical condition, thereby involving multiple clinical decisions, each with its own associated cost and consequence uncertainties. In addition, the degree of sophistication required to factor in the cost-effectiveness of implementation strategies has seldom, if ever, been addressed. Thus, cost impact assessments on guidelines may be of less value to policy makers than they suppose.

Whilst such presentations might be of interest to a guideline development group, their use needs to be handled with care. Cost impact analyses are potentially problematic since they may be perceived to take the focus away from improving individual treatment decisions: clinicians and patients may perceive that 'affordability' rather than 'values' underpins the guideline recommendations, potentially discrediting the guideline medium. However, members of guideline groups might perceive a cost impact assessment to be important at a local level. For example, it may be helpful to know how much a new screening programme will cost, organised at various levels (such as the general practitioner or primary care trust) where delivery issues and implementation are seen as integral to the recommendations.

An example in mental health: use of antidepressants in primary care

A guideline to address the initial management of depression using antidepressants in primary care was developed by the North of England Guideline Development Group during 1996–97. Its brief was to produce evidence-based recommendations on the primary care management of depression with antidepressants, reflecting effective and cost-effective care. The detailed findings have been published.[7,8] A shortened presentation of the process is provided, although it should be recognised that the evidence is historically (rather than currently) correct and the recommendations are thus illustrative. The purpose is to provide a brief example of how the attributes build together to inform the guideline development group's understanding. The guideline development group was composed of five general practitioners, two psychiatrists, one pharmaceutical advisor, one health service manager, two health service researchers, and a small-group leader.

Background

Antidepressants are the mainstay treatment of depression in English primary care. In 1995, approximately one million person-years of treatment were provided at a purchase cost of £160 million. Costs were increasing dramatically as newer (and more expensive) antidepressants received greater use (Figures 3.1 and 3.2). In particular, there was considerable uncertainty about the appropriate use of newer selective serotonin reuptake inhibitors (SSRIs) in terms of their benefits, costs and safety. These SSRIs cost five to six times more than traditional tricyclic antidepressants, although it was argued they might not increase overall healthcare costs.

Trial evidence

The review found good trial evidence addressing the short-term relative efficacy and tolerability of the various groups of antidepressants in the first-line treatment of depression. There was some debate in the group about the relevance of the predominantly secondary care population in trials to a primary care guideline: the group had to come to an explicit opinion about the relevance of these studies. Tricyclic antidepressants appeared slightly more efficacious than SSRIs or related drugs, although

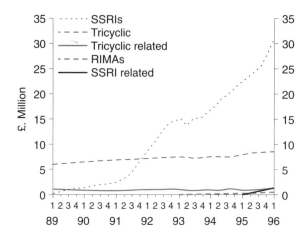

Figure 3.1: GP-prescribed antidepressants in England: cost, quarterly, 1989–1996.

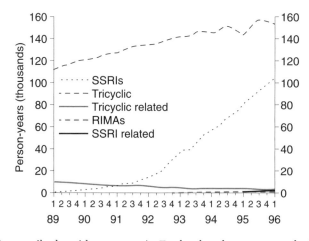

Figure 3.2: GP-prescribed antidepressants in England: volume, quarterly 1989–1996.

this effect was of uncertain practical importance. SSRIs and related drugs were slightly better tolerated than tricyclic antidepressants, as measured by reducing the risk of drop-out in trials. The median range of follow-up was six weeks in the trials.

Epidemiological evidence

The guideline development group voiced concerns about the relative safety of different classes of antidepressants. Accidental or deliberate poisoning would be more common with more toxic drugs and traumatic injury could follow from inappropriate day-time sedation. These events are rare and were not captured in trials. Previously published toxicity indices for antidepressants had been developed too early to provide reliable estimates for newer drugs. Consequently new research was conducted to match mortality-by-cause with volume of drug treatment.[9]

Poisoning fatality data associated with antidepressants for England and Wales for three years (1993–95) were combined with volume of anti-depressant use data for the same period to estimate death rates associated with specific antidepressants. Interpreting estimated death rates requires care: higher death rates might be explained by trends in the use of certain drugs with more severely depressed and co-morbid patient groups as well as underlying pharmacological toxicity. This analysis demonstrated both the rarity of fatal overdose and the large range of rates associated with individual antidepressants. Overall, one fatality was expected for about every 3000 patient-years of treatment (Table 3.1). However, tricyclic antidepressants (excluding lofepramine) linked with cardiovascular toxi-city were associated with a higher than average fatality rate. SSRIs, as a group, were found to be relatively safe, with one fatality for every 100,000 patient-years of treatment. One second-generation tricyclic antidepressant appeared atypical: lofepramine featured a fatality rate similar to the SSRIs of one fatality for every 59,000 patient-years of treatment.

Fatal poisonings were categorised according to whether single or multi-ple substances were ingested. Multiple ingestion involved taking other medicinal substances as well as an antidepressant and so these data were more difficult to interpret. Nearly 70% of all antidepressant-associated poisoning fatalities involved a single-ingested antidepressant. Fatalities were also grouped as accidental, deliberate or poisoning of unknown intent. Since only 15% were recorded as accidental, the guideline

Table 3.1: Fatality toxicity associated with antidepressants.

	Single substance death rate		Single and multiple substance death rate	
	DR*	95%CI[†]	DR	95%CI
Overall	0.339	0.328 to 0.349	0.492	0.479 to 0.505
Sub-groups				
SSRIs[‡]	0.010	0.006 to 0.013	0.041	0.034 to 0.048
Lofepramine	0.017	0.010 to 0.025	0.062	0.047 to 0.076
Tricyclic and related[§]	0.577	0.559 to 0.595	0.808	0.787 to 0.830

* Death rate (DR) by fatal poisoning and associated with named antidepressants, per 1000 person-years of treatment.
[†] 95% Confidence intervals associated with each drug were calculated as DR±1.96SE, where the standard error (SE) was estimated as $[p(1-p)/n]^{1/2}$ using the number of treatment episodes (n) and probability (p) of a fatal poisoning. The average duration of a treatment episode was assumed to be 3 months, thus treatment episodes equal patient-years of treatment multiplied by four.
[‡] Includes: citalopram, fluoxetine, fluvoxamine, paroxetine and sertraline.
[§] Includes all tricyclic and related antidepressants except lofepramine.

development group were uncertain whether fatalities could be significantly reduced by a policy of wide-scale switching to less toxic antidepressants.

Cost-effectiveness modelling

Some cases of antidepressant poisoning may not result in a fatality but be severe enough to require hospitalisation. Additionally some hospitalisations due to accidents may arise from inappropriate sedation, although in some patients sedation is an intended treatment effect. National data exist on the total number of hospitalisations for poisoning and trauma and it was possible to make high and low estimates of the number of these attributable to tricyclic antidepressant use.

The guideline development group developed two scenarios, optimistic and conservative, to explore the merits of using SSRI and lofepramine antidepressants instead of other tricyclics. These provide a profile of the likely consequences in changes in GP and outpatient visits, and psychiatric, poisoning and accident admissions alongside the likely costs. Consequently, the incremental cost-effectiveness of using lofepramine ranged from £60,000 to £520,000 per life saved and subsequently switching from lofepramine to an SSRI was estimated to cost from £7.1 million to £60 million per life saved.

The overall strength of evidence was low, reflecting the needs of the model to incorporate a range of observational data sources. Potentially economic models could always feature poorly under any evidence grading scheme but judgement is required. If a model structure is clinically and epidemiologically valid and verifiable and its findings are robust, with key parameters based on high-quality evidence, then overall a high grade may be assigned and new evidence grading schemes are being developed to reflect this.

Guideline development group findings

The recommendations and supporting evidence statements of the North of England Guideline Development Group are reproduced in Box 3.4.

Conclusions

Modern guidelines have to meet the informational needs not just of clinicians but also of patients and carers and be consistent with national policy aims. While not all patients may wish to participate in the clinical decisions that affect them, clinicians should inform and enable patients to participate in decision making to the extent that they are willing and able. The role of economic analysis within clinical guidelines is to direct

Box 3.4: Recommendations and supporting evidence of the North of England Guideline Development Group

- As they represent the most cost-effective option, tricyclic antidepressants should be used as the routine first-line drug treatment for depression in primary care.
  - Tricyclic antidepressants appear slightly more efficacious than SSRIs or related drugs, although this effect is of uncertain practical importance.
  - SSRIs and related drugs are slightly better tolerated than tricyclic antidepressants, reducing the risk of drop-out by about 4% during 6 weeks of treatment in double-blind randomised trials.
- If the toxic effects of the older tricyclic antidepressants are perceived to be a problem, for example in a patient who has previously taken a drug overdose, then lofepramine is a more cost-effective choice than an SSRI.
  - There is a substantial range of toxicity associated with different antidepressants as currently used in primary care. The SSRIs and lofepramine are associated with the smallest risk of fatal poisoning.
  - A general policy of switching from tricyclics to SSRIs does not appear cost-effective. Where the toxic effects of tricyclic antidepressants give cause for concern, substitution with lofepramine appears relatively cost-effective.
- The choice of antidepressant should be based on individual patient factors. These would include:
  - the desirability or otherwise of sedation or other effects associated with a particular drug
  - previous response to a particular drug
  - co-morbid psychiatric or medical conditions
  - concurrent drug therapy.
- The dose of tricyclic antidepressants should be titrated up to the doses used in the clinical trials.
- Lower doses should be used initially in older patients.
- If patient compliance is a concern, tricyclic antidepressants can be given in a once-daily dosage.
- When faced with a patient not responding to first-line drug therapy reasonable options are:
  - review the diagnosis
  - check compliance with drug therapy
  - consider a change in drug treatment
  - consider the potential contribution of maintaining factors (e.g. co-morbidity, poor housing, etc.)
  - consider referral to a psychiatrist.

SSRI: selective serotonin reuptake inhibitor

decision making more consistently towards a better use of scarce resources. Williams suggested that 'The immediate task of health economists is to get our notions of efficiency and fairness in the distribution of the benefits of healthcare so deeply embedded in the clinical consciousness that they come to be thought of as wholly within the realm of clinical autonomy'.[10] This is realistic if those who develop clinical practice guidelines both understand the realities of clinical care and thoughtfully engage its audience in the social valuation of healthcare.

Acknowledgements

This chapter is based on the contents of the UK NHS R&D Health Technology Assessment Programme Report: Eccles M and Mason J (2001) How to develop cost-conscious guidelines. *Health Technol Assess.* 5(16).

References

1   Eddy DM (1992) *A Manual for Assessing Health Practices and Designing Practice Policies: the explicit approach.* American College of Physicians, Philadelphia, PA.

2   Institute of Medicine (1992) *Guidelines for Clinical Practice: from development to use.* National Academy Press, Washington, DC.

3   Williams A (1995) How should information on cost effectiveness influence clinical practice? In: T Delamothe (ed.) *Outcomes into Clinical Practice.* BMJ Books, London, pp. 99–107.

4   Mason J, Eccles M, Freemantle N *et al.* (1999) A framework for incorporating cost-effectiveness in evidence based clinical practice guidelines. *Health Policy.* 47: 37–52.

5   Freemantle N and Mason JM (1997) Publication bias in clinical trials and economic analyses. *Pharmacoeconomics.* 12(1): 10–16.

6   Mason JM (1997) The generalisability of pharmacoeconomic studies. *Pharmacoeconomics.* 11: 503–14.

7   North of England Evidence Based Guideline Development Project (1998) *The Choice of Antidepressants for Depression in Primary Care.* University of Newcastle, Centre for Health Services Research, Newcastle.

8   Eccles M, Freemantle N and Mason JM for the North of England Guideline Development Group (1999) The choice of antidepressants for depression in primary care. *Fam Pract.* 16: 103–11.

9   Mason J, Freemantle N and Eccles M (2000) Fatal toxicity associated with antidepressant use in primary care. *Br J Gen Pract.* 50: 366–70.

10 Williams A (1988) Health economics: the end of clinical freedom? *BMJ.* 297: 1183–6.

Chapter 4

The legal status of clinical practice guidelines

Brian S Hurwitz

'Guidelines have no defined legal position. However, any doctor not fulfilling the standards and quality of care in the appropriate treatment that are set out in these Clinical Guidelines, will have this taken into account if, for any reason, consideration of their performance in this clinical area is undertaken.'

Department of Health (1999)[1]

'Guidelines are no substitute for expert evidence about acceptable practice. Compliance with well-recognised guidelines is likely to exculpate (exonerate). Deviation from well-recognised guidelines may be Bolam-defensible.'

C Foster, Barrister (2002)[2]

The authority and standing of clinical practice guidelines were first recognised to be important professional and legal issues by Plato in the 4th century BC. Plato was interested in the difference between human skills grounded in practical expertise and those based solely upon following instructions or obeying rules. The pervasive influence of guidelines on the practice of modern medicine and the varied approaches to guideline development that exist, with consequent effects on clinical practice guideline quality, ensure that the legal status of guidelines continues to be debated today.

Plato invented the following thought-experiment to explore the matter. Doctors were to be stripped of their clinical freedom – 'no longer allowed unchecked authority' – and were to form themselves into councils to determine majority views about how best to practise medicine in all situations. The deliberations and majority decisions of such panels (composed of clinical and non-clinical members) were to be codified and published in order 'to dictate the ways in which the treatment of the sick was to be practised'.[3] Plato viewed the hallmarks of expertise to be flexible responsiveness and improvisatory ability – aspects of medical practice still recognised today – which he believed would be endangered by the use of guidelines.[3] However effective healthcare by guideline turned out to be

– and Plato was prepared to concede its potential – such care would constitute a debased form of practice, because guidelines, he believed, presupposed standardised treatments for average patients rather than customised treatments for particular patients. Also the knowledge and analysis that go into the creation of guidelines are not rooted in the mental processes of clinicians, but in the minds of guideline developers distant from the consultation. Very similar concerns continue to trouble present-day clinicians (*see* Box 4.1).

Box 4.1

'There is a fear that in the absence of evidence clearly applicable to the case in hand a clinician might be forced by guidelines to make use of evidence which is only doubtfully relevant, generated perhaps in a different grouping of patients in another country and some other time and using a similar but not identical treatment. This is . . . to use evidence in the manner of the fabled drunkard who searched under the street lamp for his door key because that is where the light was, even though he had dropped the key somewhere else.'[4]

J Grimley Evans, Professor of Geriatric Medicine,
University of Oxford

'The extent to which guidelines depend on opinion is disturbing for anyone who believes they should be evidence based. Guidelines are evidence filtered through opinion. The opinion is crucial – but whose opinion should it be? The NICE committee is made up of a variety of experts in different disciplines who take specific advice from a small number of specialists in the relevant field. These specialists may or may not hold an opinion widely shared by their (equally expert) colleagues.'[5]

J Hampton, Professor of Cardiology, University of Nottingham

In Plato's view, once a profession committed itself to providing healthcare through guidelines (a position now demanded by the UK government),[6,7] he could see no alternative but to ensure compliance with them, even if this entailed resorting to legal action. Such guidelines, he believed, would have to be understood almost as clinical laws. Once expertise resides no longer within the patient's clinician but is represented instead in guidelines, corruption of, or deviation from, such guidelines would result in medical treatments being grounded in personal whim or quackery.

Plato's reference to the legal arena was remarkable in its prescience. Only comparatively recently have guidelines begun to feature in modern-day healthcare regulations and in case law.[8–12] Today, the General Medical

Council advises clinical teams 'normally to use recommended clinical guidelines'.[13]

Guidelines and legislation

Legislation in Europe and the USA has harnessed guidelines to a variety of healthcare regulatory tasks.[14,15] An example in the UK is the Human Fertilisation and Embryology Act 1990, which established a regulatory authority (HFEA) empowered to develop guidelines.[16] The HFEA initially decided to restrict to three the number of fertilised eggs that can legally be placed in a woman's uterus during treatment by *in vitro* fertilisation (IVF). The Authority later reduced this number to two. The mandatory nature of the HFEA's guidance on this matter in the event of transgression is made plain by enforceable penalties, including revocation of the licence to practise IVF. The HFEA's 'guidance' on this is backed by Parliamentary authority and carries the force of a prescriptive legal rule.

In France, mandatory practice guidelines introduced under a 1993 statute, Loi Teulade 93-8, cover investigations, prescribing and certain medical procedures. Initially developed by the social security administration responsible for reimbursing private practitioners and the doctors' unions, guideline development has now been taken over by an independent organisation, the Agence Nationale pour le Développement de l'Evaluation Médicale. Once published, the guidelines constitute an enforceable agreement between doctors and the social security administration.[17,18]

Standards of medical care

The legally required standard of medical treatment a doctor generally owes to a patient derives in the UK from the case of *Bolam v Friern Hospital Management Committee* (1957). In the words of the judge of this case, 'The test is the standard of the ordinary skilled man exercising and professing to have that special skill'.[19] The judge in Bolam recognised that there could be two or more schools of thought regarding proper medical treatment. Therefore, doctors can usually rebut a charge of negligence if they have acted in conformity with a body of other responsible doctors.[19]

Expert testimony helps the courts to ascertain what is accepted and proper practice in specific cases, ensuring that professionally generated standards derived from real clinical situations are generally applied by the courts, rather than standards enunciated in the rhetoric of clinical practice guidelines. In *Cranley v Medical Board of Western Australia* (1990) an Australian GP stood accused of misconduct because he had prescribed injectable diazepam to heroin addicts, contrary to the Australian National Methadone Guidelines. He was initially found guilty of 'infamous and improper conduct', but after hearing of a minority medical opinion supporting treatment of opiate addicts within the harm reduction framework followed by Dr Cranley, the Supreme Court of Western Australia upheld his appeal.[20]

As a norm, the Bolam test is supposed to represent an aggregate of individual clinical judgements informed by scientific evidence and professional experience. Its advantages are held to be that it takes account of evolving standards of care and is a professionally led (though legally imposed) standard. It allows for differences of opinion and is sufficiently broadly expressed to encompass medical practice that is predominantly scientific or as much a craft as a science.

Box 4.2: Negligence

Medical negligence is a composite finding comprising three essential elements. The complainant, formerly the plaintiff, the person bringing the action, must show that:

1 the defendant doctor owed the complainant a duty of care, and
2 the doctor breached this duty of care by failing to provide the required standard of medical care, and
3 this failure actually caused the plaintiff harm – a harm that was both foreseeable and reasonably avoidable.

Clinical guidelines could influence the manner in which the courts establish the second element of this composite.

However, unlike the tests of negligence adopted in other common law jurisdictions, such as Canada (where the test is based on 'that degree of care and skill which could *reasonably be expected* of a normal prudent practitioner of the same experience and standing'),[21] the Bolam test appears to be more a 'state of the art' descriptive test about what *is* done in practice than a normative test of what *ought* to be done. Under Bolam, widespread adoption of guidelines could result in guideline-informed care becoming viewed as the customary norm, with departure from guidelines then being seen as *prima facie* evidence of a case to answer.[22,23]

A leading UK barrister has concluded that the effects of guidelines and evidence-based medicine together are that 'many areas of medicine and surgery, which attract the attention of civil litigators, are or will be governed by clinical guidelines. Increasingly, it will be possible to plead just one particular type of negligence: "Failing to follow guideline X"'.[2] Given the poor quality of many clinical practice guidelines currently in circulation, this consequence should be guarded against (*see* Box 4.3).[24] Some guideline quality markers may be a crude indication of overall guideline quality, but the potential for poor-quality guidelines to influence the legal standard by which a doctor is judged is compounded by the failure of the courts generally to call expert witnesses to scrutinise the robustness and quality of guidelines.[25,26]

Box 4.3: Quality indicators of clinical guidelines published in peer review journals over a 10-year period

Of 431 clinical guidelines published in English, listed in MEDLINE and produced by specialty societies between January 1988 and July 1998, 88% were found to give no information on the searches used to retrieve relevant published studies, 67% failed to report any description of the type of stakeholders involved in guideline development or use, and 82% provided no explicit grading of the strength of recommendations.[24]

The Bolam test in the UK operates on a case-by-case basis. Lord Woolf, the Lord Chief Justice of England, speaking extra-judicially to the Royal College of Physicians of London about legal standards of care, said:

> 'The general approach of the courts is to apply the standards that the medical profession adopts. Thus we judge whether there has been negligence in the treatment of a patient by asking whether or not the medical treatment, which is the subject of complaint, accords with standards which *any* recognised section of the medical profession regards as acceptable . . . By adopting this standard the courts have managed to hold the balance fairly between the interests of the patient and the interest of the profession. By striking the right balance, the courts reduce the risk of proper medical practice being undermined by fear of litigation and recognise the need for compensation to be paid where treatment is of an unacceptable standard.'[27]

Hitherto, the main justification for judicial reliance upon customary care standards has been the belief that technical medical matters are beyond the detailed knowledge of judges and lay people and are best left to 'experts'. Since guidelines offer doctors and patients explicit examples of standards of care articulated in considerable detail for use in specific clinical circumstances, they could be thought to remove the need for expert testimony in court, as the courts would have direct access to relevant standards from guidelines.[22,24]

However, guidelines may not in fact reflect customary standards of care at all. Indeed, some appear designed to hasten the incorporation of research findings into routine practice.[28] This inevitably challenges the law's use of a customary care standard that does little to narrow gaps between everyday clinical practices and evidence-based practice. In an evidence-linked era, Bolam may be thought to demand too little to encourage higher standards of care. Condemned as 'a blot on English medical law', the Bolam test has been disparaged as the result of undue judicial deference to medical opinion. But despite no longer being as influential as it once was, Bolam has not yet been superseded in the UK by a legal standard entirely determined without reference to a responsible body of medical practitioners (*see* Box 4.4).[29,31]

Box 4.4: Guidelines are no substitute for expert evidence

Guidelines could be introduced to a court by an expert witness as evidence of accepted and customary standards of care, but they cannot be introduced as a substitute for expert testimony. Courts are unlikely to adopt standards of care advocated in clinical guidelines as legal 'gold standards', because the mere fact that a guideline exists does not of itself establish that compliance with it is reasonable in the circumstances or that non-compliance is negligent. 'Guidelines are no substitute for expert evidence about acceptable practice. Compliance with well-recognised guidelines is likely to exculpate (exonerate). Deviation from well-recognised guidelines may be Bolam-defensible.'

C Foster, Barrister (2002)[2]

Author or sponsor liability

That bias might creep into guideline development has been a concern in France, where complaints have been laid before the Fraud Squad alleging improper conduct by participants in the French guidelines programme.[17] It is also a concern of the American Medical Association (AMA), which believes that 'bad faith claims could be lodged against developers who stand to benefit from the content of a guideline and who design results to comport with desired cost containment goals'.[30]

In the USA, the AMA has outlined the scenarios which could found a claim against guideline developers or sponsors in the event of faulty guidelines being associated with patient harm (*see* Box 4.5). These include negligence in 'analysing or interpreting data, or translating data into a guideline, ignoring well-known and scientifically valid data, and utilising data that were known, or should have been known, to be insufficient or faulty'.[30] But to date, no cases have arisen in either US or UK jurisdictions in which the courts have been required to decide whether guideline authors were liable for incorrect or misleading statements (*see* Box 4.6).[2,30-4]

Box 4.5: AMA advice to US guideline developers

The AMA believes developers of guidelines should 'assume that their research methodology and resulting conclusions will subsequently be subject to legal review and to proceed with the assumption that they may be challenged in court. In keeping with this approach, the guidelines' underlying methodology, supporting research, recommendations, and conclusions should be fully documented and preserved for inspection by others at a later time.'[30]

Box 4.6: Author/sponsor liability

'While an action could be taken against a clinician for not keeping up to date, a College is probably not actionable, as it would be difficult to show it owes a duty or obligation directly to the patient.'

NHS Executive (1996)[37]

In non-medical spheres, UK courts have decided similar questions where people have suffered economic loss by relying upon written statements of advice.[35] However, the general position in the UK is that there can be no duty of care between the author of a document or book and its myriad potential readers, unless the authors could foresee that their written advice would be directly communicated to a reader, who would have little choice but to rely upon it without independent enquiry. Such advice would need to possess quite extraordinary authority for doctors to be expected to follow clinical practice guidelines without further enquiry.[36]

The status of advice offered by guidelines should be made as clear as possible to clinicians. For example, the prefatory statement in the NICE guidelines on *Core Interventions in the Treatment and Management of Schizophrenia in Primary and Secondary Care* reads:

'This guidance represents the view of the Institute, which was arrived at after careful consideration of the evidence available. Health professionals are expected to take it fully into account when exercising their clinical judgement. The guidance does not, however, over-ride the individual responsibility of health professionals to make decisions appropriate to the circumstances of the individual patient, in consultation with the patient and/or guardian or carer.'[38]

Though this seems like a disclaimer, the authors emphasise that users of the guideline are expected to behave as learned intermediaries, exercising customary clinical discretion and consulting other sources of relevant information.

Discretion

Some health service lawyers have commented that as guidelines receive increasing acceptance in the clinical community, acting in accordance with a clinical practice guideline could be viewed as acceptable medical practice *per se*. However, guidelines can create a false sense of consensus, can mask or underplay controversy and may rapidly become out of date as a result of new findings. Most guidelines face more or less well-grounded degrees of dissent most of the time. For example, in 2003, the *Drugs and Therapeutics Bulletin* systematically reviewed the role of intravenous magnesium administration in the treatment of severe asthma and concluded that:

> 'The current British Guideline on the Management of Asthma, published jointly by the British Thoracic Society and the Scottish Intercollegiate Guidelines Network, suggests that a single i.v. dose of magnesium sulphate should be used for the treatment of patients with acute severe asthma.[39] However, the available data are weak and conflicting and do not justify this unlicensed use of the drug.'[40]

In general, doctors are expected to use appropriate clinical discretion when deciding upon medical treatment and the courts continue to place the testimony of expert witnesses about what constitutes reasonable practice above the recommendations of prestigious works of reference (*see* Box 4.4). Even where a guideline has been laid down as a legal standard, courts require sensible discretion to be used in its appropriate application.[41]

In administrative law the essence of discretion is 'a readiness to deal with each case on its merits'.[42] The NHS Executive acknowledges that when endorsed by prestigious professional bodies or even commended by the NHS Executive:

> '. . . clinical guidelines can still only assist the practitioner; they cannot be used to mandate, authorise or outlaw treatment options. Regardless of the strength of the evidence, it will remain the responsibility of the practising clinicians to interpret their application . . . It would be wholly inappropriate for clinical

guidelines to be used as a means of coercion of the individual clinician, by managers and senior professionals.'[37]

Rigid, uncritical adherence to guidelines is not the formal, administrative or managerial expectation in the NHS. Translation of precepts into action involves interpretation,[43] as emphasised in guidelines on the treatment of hypertension produced by the World Health Organization:

> 'Guidelines should provide extensive, critical, and well-balanced information on benefits and limitations of the various diagnostic and therapeutic interventions so that the physician may exert the most careful judgement in individual cases.'[44]

Concern remains, however, that guidelines could erode clinical abilities, diminish clinical judgement and reduce medical practice to 'cookbook medicine' and the thoughtless activities of physician automata.[45] In the USA, tensions surfacing between treatment protocols and doctors' clinical judgement have led the courts to rule that clinicians may not claim as a defence to negligence that their clinical judgement has been corrupted by guidelines.[46]

Although some judgements required of doctors in discrete areas of medicine can be more or less explicitly specified, this should not be thought to reduce clinical judgements to nothing other than 'decisional algebra', which can be objectified in expert systems, algorithms, protocols or guidelines. Clinical practice frequently involves judgements about complex individual circumstances in the context of different degrees of uncertainty. Medical decision making depends on opinionated assessments that are grounded in knowledge of appropriate scientific findings, which are informed by clinical experience and take account of patients' wishes. Such decisions are not simple transductions of input information resulting in output decisions. Clinical judgements frequently go beyond explicit input information, adding considerations of feeling, attitude and value to the output.[47] As one distinguished professor of cardiology has expressed: 'Treatment can depend on something as subtle and unquantifiable as the glint in a patient's eye'.[48] Applying guidelines to individual care is always likely to require judgement, even when recommendations are properly evidence linked.[49] Sir Michael Rawlins, the Chairman of NICE, accepts that: 'No guideline can cover 100 per cent, because people vary. It's up to the doctor or other health professional to decide when the guideline is no longer applicable and what to do in its place'.[50]

The implication of Sir Michael's view – that some clinical decisions taken in situations covered by guidelines may quite properly deviate from them – does not detract from the advice issued by Vivienne Nathanson, head of the Science, Ethics and Policy Unit of the BMA (and endorsed by Sir Michael Rawlins[50]) that doctors should record treatment decisions in patients' notes in ways that 'show that they have considered the guidelines'.[51]

NICE and guidelines

How, if at all, does the arrival of the National Institute for Clinical Excellence alter the legal status of guidelines? NICE was set up to give guidance to the NHS as a whole, to the government and ultimately to patients, in several areas of healthcare, including the creation of clinical practice guidelines.[52] According to the DoH memorandum setting out the groundrules under which NICE operates, the Institute is required to follow a transparent and well-structured process, giving appropriate interested parties the opportunity to submit evidence and to comment on draft conclusions. The memorandum conceptualises the Department's view of the legal status of NICE guidance in the following terms:

> 'All guidance must be fully reasoned and written in terms which makes clear that it is guidance. Guidance for clinicians does not over-ride their professional responsibility to make the appropriate decision in the circumstances of the individual patient, in consultation with the patient or guardian/carer and in the light of any locally agreed policies. Similarly, guidance to NHS trusts and commissioners must make clear that it does not take away their discretion under administrative law to take account of individual circumstances.'[52]

This status was not altered by the introduction, in January 2002, of a statutory obligation on NHS organisations to fund NICE-appraised treatments. However, NICE has also been charged with ensuring that the implications of its recommendations are transmitted to National Service Frameworks and related quality of care initiatives, such as the following NHS information and advice channels: PRODIGY guidelines, the National electronic Library for Health, protocols used by NHS Direct and NHS walk-in centres, any material for patients produced by NHS Direct Online.[52] NICE is therefore structurally and strategically positioned to be at the hub of a series of influential mechanisms designed to facilitate implementation of guidance. How realistic, therefore, is the Department's simultaneously held view that NICE-approved guidance should not be thought to under-cut or over-ride clinicians' professional responsibility to make appropriate decisions in the circumstances of the individual patient?

A 1999 legal case, which arose from a desire to limit a drug's use within the NHS, has clearly indicated that the language in which advice is couched can significantly influence how guidance is likely to be interpreted. Its language can also bear on the lawfulness of its guidance. In *R v Secretary of State for Health ex parte Pfizer Ltd* (May 1999)[53] the lawfulness of a

Health Service Circular (1998/158)[54] dated 16 September 1998 was challenged in the High Court. Although the circular in question contained the heading '*Material which is for guidance only and aims to share good practice*' the judge ruled that the circular was advice in presentation only. In substance and effect it was a direction which unlawfully curtailed the clinical discretion of UK general practitioners – a discretion, moreover, which has statutory underpinning[55]: 'The problem with the circular is that the advice was given in a manner which meant that GPs would inevitably regard it as over-riding their professional judgement . . . '.[53]

The case highlights the potential power of a clinical practice guideline agency such as NICE. On the one hand, the model hitherto construed to characterise physician–guideline relationships posits doctors as free agents, capable of appropriately taking advantage of authoritative guidance without entering into a relationship of professional *reliance* upon guideline guidance. But as the analysis of Health Service Circular 1998/158 indicates, executive implementation of authoritative guidance carries with it a danger that guidance can all too easily be packaged as (and therefore mistaken for) instructions. If this happens, it will significantly undermine the ability of clinicians to act as their own 'master editors' of advisory information, able to modify and blend guideline advice with their own experience in the context of the advice of local treatment policies. It may be that this model of practice is now a diminishing ideal, one perhaps applicable only to specialists in their own field of expertise, who have both the appropriate depth of experience and knowledge to avoid over-reliance on clinical practice guidelines.[5,48]

Conclusions

Despite stirrings afoot to replace the customary Bolam standard of medical care with a normative standard that would be more susceptible to determination without reference to a professional body of medical opinion, there appears to be no managerial or legal expectation in the UK that doctors should automatically follow guidelines. Clinical practice guidelines are not generally credited by the courts with a special 'self-evident' status and guidelines currently play a subservient role to that of the expert witness in court proceedings.[34] The only published study of actual guideline use in litigation revealed that in the USA guidelines play 'a relevant or pivotal role in the proof of negligence' in less than 7% of US malpractice actions.[56]

Nevertheless, clinical practice guidelines look set to become more influential in both the way doctors practise and the manner in which they are to be held accountable. The GMC has announced a general expectation that doctors 'will normally follow guidelines'[13] and the courts tend to look to the GMC in matters of ethical guidance.[57] The creation of

NICE, with its dual role of developing authoritative guidelines and of disseminating them through official NHS channels, means its guidelines are likely to be credited with a distinctive title to be believed from a legal point of view.[58,59]

In future, adherence to NICE guidelines which allegedly are associated with patient harm is therefore likely to exonerate the defendant doctor, unless it can be shown that the guidelines followed are faulty or inappropriately or unthinkingly applied in a particular case. Deviation from NICE guidelines is likely to inculpate a defendant unless he or she can show that the guidelines not followed are faulty or face sufficient counter-evidence to justify a body of responsible doctors deviating from them.[60]

Clinical discretion remains at the core of what it means to be a doctor exercising professional judgement. But discretion in the circumstances of modern healthcare is characterised by many potentially competing pressures – from patient choice, clinical practice guidelines, targets, costs and incentives. The sort of discretion to be exercised in the use of guidelines should probably be understood to be different from that exercised in using other decision-making aids, such as textbooks, lecture notes or expert systems. Guidelines are 'standardised specifications of care'[51] which are inherently designed to constrain clinical discretion in ways never envisaged by the authors of textbooks.

But against the increased constraint on clinical discretion that guidelines undoubtedly exercise, and unlike the consensus guidelines envisaged by Plato, modern-day evidence-linked clinical practice guidelines seek to make transparent the strengths, weaknesses and relevance of research evidence to clinical care. Such guidelines generally take years to prepare and for most of their life span they co-exist with evidence that is frequently thought to challenge aspects of their guidance. In addition, many guidelines of poorer quality remain in circulation.[61] Guidelines cited in court proceedings should therefore be scrutinised by experts for their quality, validity and currency, and for their relevance and applicability to the case in question.

References

1 Department of Health (1999) *Drug Misuse and Dependence – Guidelines on clinical management.* Department of Health, London.
2 Foster C (2002) Civil procedure, trial issues and clinical guidelines. In: J Tingle and C Foster (eds) *Clinical Guidelines: law, policy and practice.* Cavendish Publishing, London.
3 Annas J and Waterfield R (eds) (1995) *Plato. Statesman.* Cambridge University Press, Cambridge.
4 Grimley Evans J (1995) Evidence-based and evidence-biased medicine. *Age and Ageing.* **24**: 461–3.

5   Hampton JR (2003) Guidelines – for the obedience of fools and the guidance of wise men? *Clin Med.* **3**: 279–84.

6   Secretary of State for Health (1997) *The New NHS: modern, dependable*. HMSO, London.

7   Department of Health (2001) *A Commitment to Quality: quest for excellence*. HMSO, London.

8   Loveday v Renton and Wellcome Foundation Ltd (QBD) (1990) 1 *Med Law Reports*: 117–204.

9   Re W (A minor) (1992) 3 *Weekly Law Reports*: 758–82.

10 Ratty v Haringey HA (1994) 5 *Med Law Reports*: 413.

11 Airedale NHS Trust v Bland (Guardian ad litem) (1993) 1 *All England Reports*: 821–96.

12 Early v Newham Health Authority (1994) 5 *Med Law Reports*. 215–17.

13 General Medical Council (1998) *Maintaining Good Medical Practice*. GMC, London.

14 Ministry of Justice (1993) Directie Voorlichting: Act amending Act on the Disposal of the Dead. *Staatsblad*: 643. Cited in: van der Wal G and Dillman RJ (1994) Euthanasia in the Netherlands. *BMJ.* **308**: 1346–9.

15 Public Law 101–239, the Omnibus Reconciliation Act (1989) In: M Field and K Lohr (eds) *Clinical Practice Guidelines: directions for a new program*. Institute of Medicine, National Academy Press, Washington, DC.

16 Human Fertilisation and Embryology Authority (1991) *Code of Practice CH(91)5*. HFEA, London.

17 Maisonneuve H, Codier H, Durocher A *et al.* (1997) The French clinical guidelines and medical references programme: development of 48 guidelines for private practice over a period of 18 months. *J Eval Clin Pract.* **3**: 3–13.

18 Durand-Zaleski I, Colin C and Blum-Boisgard C (1997) An attempt to save money using mandatory practice guidelines in France. *BMJ.* **315**: 943–6.

19 Bolam v Friern Hospital Management Committee (1957) 2 *All England Reports*: 118–28.

20 Cranley v Medical Board of Western Australia (Sup Ct WA) (1992) 3 *Med Law Reports*: 94–113.

21 Crits v Sylvester (1956) *OR*: 132, *1 DLR* (2d): 502, affirmed (1956) *SCR*: 991, 5 *DLR* (2d): 601.

22 Harpwood V (1994) NHS reform, audit, protocols and standards of care. *Med Law Int.* **1**: 241–59.

23 Stern K (1995) Clinical guidelines and negligence liability. In: M Deighan and S Hitch (eds) *Clinical Effectiveness: from guidelines to cost effective practice*. Earlybrave Publications, Brentwood.

24 Grilli R, Magrini N, Penna A *et al.* (2000) Practice guidelines developed by specialty societies: the need for a critical appraisal. *Lancet.* **355**: 103–6.

25 Pierre v Marshall (1993) AJ No. 1095.

26 McDonagh RJ and Hurwitz B (2003) Lying in the bed we've made: reflections on some unintended consequences of clinical practice guidelines in the courts. *J Obstet Gynaecol Can.* **25**(2): 139–43.

27 The Right Honorable Lord Woolf (1997) Medics, lawyers and the courts. *J Roy Coll Phys Lond.* **31**: 686–93.

28 Haines A and Jones R (1994) Implementing findings of research. *BMJ.* **308**: 1488–92.

29 Bolitho v City & Hackney Health Authority (1997) **3** *Weekly Law Reports*: 1151–61.

30 Schantz SJ (1999) Developing and implementing clinical practice guidelines: legal aspects. AMA, Chicago, pp. 16, 19. Cites Rosoff AJ (1995) The role of clinical practice guidelines in healthcare reform. *Health Matrix*. **5**: 369, 390.

31 Hurwitz B (2003) Medico-legal issues. In: R Jones, N Britten, L Culpepper *et al.* (eds) *Oxford Textbook of Primary Medical Care*, Vol. 1. Oxford University Press, Oxford, pp. 598–604.

32 Whitty P, Eccles M, Woolf SH *et al.* (2003) Using and developing clinical guidelines. In: R Jones, N Britten, L Culpepper *et al.* (eds) *Oxford Textbook of Primary Medical Care*, Vol. 1. Oxford University Press, Oxford, pp. 477–84.

33 Newdick C (1995) *Who Should We Treat?* Clarendon Press, Oxford.

34 Hurwitz B (1998) *Clinical Guidelines and the Law: negligence, discretion and judgment*. Radcliffe Medical Press, Oxford.

35 Caparo Industries plc v Dickman and others (1990) **1** *All Engl Law Reports*: 568–608.

36 National Health and Medical Research Council (1995) Legal implications of guidelines. In: *Guidelines for the Development and Implementation of Clinical Guidelines*. Australian Government Publishing Service, Canberra.

37 National Health Service Executive (1996) *Clinical Guidelines*. NHSE, Leeds.

38 National Collaborating Centre for Mental Health (2002) *Core Interventions in the Treatment and Management of Schizophrenia in Primary and Secondary Care*. NICE, London.

39 Scottish Intercollegiate Guidelines Network, The British Thoracic Society (2003) British guideline on the management of asthma. *Thorax*. **58** (suppl 1): i1–94.

40 Anonymous (2003) Intravenous magnesium for acute asthma? *Drug Ther Bull*. **41**(10): 79–80.

41 McFarlane v Secretary of State for Scotland (1988) *Scottish Civil Law Reports*: 623–8.

42 Cane P (1992) *An Introduction to Administrative Law*. Clarendon Press, Oxford.

43 Hawkins K (1992) *The Uses of Discretion*. Clarendon Press, Oxford.

44 Subcommittee of WHO/ISH Mild Hypertension Liaison Committee (1993) Summary of 1993 World Health Organization – International Society of Hypertension guidelines for the management of mild hypertension. *BMJ*. **307**: 1541–6.

45 Ellwood PM (1988) Outcomes management. A technology of patient experience. *N Engl J Med*. **318**: 1549–56.

46 Wickline v California (1986) *California Reporter*. **228**: 661–7.

47 McPherson K (1990) Why do variations occur? In: TF Anderson and G Mooney (eds) *The Challenge of Medical Practice Variations*. Macmillan, London.

48 Hampton JR (2000) The National Service Framework for coronary heart disease: the emperor's new clothes. *J Roy Coll Phys Lond*. **34**: 226–30.

49 Black D (1998) The limitations of evidence. *J Roy Coll Phys London*. **32**: 23–5.

50 Quoted in: Taylor J (2003) Tough talk from the NICE man. *MedEconomics*. **November**: 44–6.

51 Quoted in: Jones J (1999) Influenza drug to undergo 'fast track' assessment by NICE. *BMJ*. **319**: 400.

52 National Health Service Executive (1999) *Health Service Circular, 176*. NHSE, Leeds.

53 R v Secretary of State for Health ex parte Pfizer Ltd (1999) Case No. CO/4934/98, High Court of Justice, Queen's Bench Division, May 1999 at 20–5.

54 National Health Service Executive (1998) *Sildenafil (Viagra). Health Service Circular, 158*. NHSE, Leeds.

55 National Health Service (General Medical Services) (1992) *Regulations SI 1992* (as amended). **635**: 83–4, 138.

56 Hyams AL, Brandenburg JA, Lipsitz SR *et al.* (1995) Practice guidelines and malpractice litigation: a two way street. *Ann Int Med.* **122**: 450–5.

57 W v Egdell (1990) Ch 359.

58 Hurwitz B (2000) Clinical guidelines, NICE products and legal liability? In: A Miles, R Hampton and B Hurwitz (eds) *NICE, CHI and the NHS Reforms: enabling excellence or imposing control?* Aesculapius Medical Press, London.

59 Samanta A, Samanta J and Gunn M (2003) Legal considerations of clinical guidelines: will NICE make a difference? *J Roy Soc Med.* **96**: 133–8.

60 Symmonds M, Matheson NJ and Harnden A (2004) Guidelines on neuraminidase inhibitors in children are not supported by evidence [letter]. *BMJ.* **328**: 227.

61 Beutler LE, Clarkin JF and Bongar B (2000) *Guidelines for the Systematic Treatment of the Depressed Patient*. Oxford University Press, Oxford.

Chapter 5

Using clinical practice guidelines

Gene Feder, Martin Eccles, Richard Grol, Chris Griffiths and Jeremy Grimshaw

The development of good guidelines does not ensure their use in practice. Lomas[1] has observed the multitude of factors that influence healthcare professionals' behaviour and this has led to increased recognition of potential barriers and facilitators to implementation at various levels: the organisation, the peer group and for the individual clinician. Therefore, to maximise the likelihood of a clinical practice guideline being used, we need coherent dissemination and implementation strategies to capitalise on known facilitators and to address identified barriers. In this chapter we discuss how healthcare organisations (e.g. hospitals, general practices) and individual clinicians can use clinical practice guidelines to improve clinical effectiveness. We suggest that there are two broad methods of effective guideline use, both of which should be planned, proactive processes. First, healthcare organisations may use guidelines as tools within planned quality improvement activities. Second, individual healthcare professionals may use guidelines as an information source for continuing professional educational development and to answer specific clinical questions arising out of their day-to-day practice.[2,3]

Using clinical guidelines within healthcare organisations

The dissemination and implementation of guidelines as part of quality improvement activities within a healthcare organisation require planning, commitment, enthusiasm and resources. Quality improvement implies a cyclical process involving priority setting, implementation, assessment of performance (using clinical audit) and further implementation.

Preparation for dissemination and implementation

Priority setting

Healthcare organisations will only be able to support the implementation of a limited number of clinical practice guidelines at any one time. Therefore, in the same way as topics for guidelines development need to be prioritised,[4] organisations need a process by which they can set and pursue their clinical priorities. These can reflect national priorities (e.g. the content of the National Service Framework (NSF) for Mental Health) or can be set at a local level by commissioners, trusts or individual general practices. Irrespective of the level at which priorities are set, explicit criteria can help guide a rational choice. A number of criteria for prioritising clinical topics have been suggested[5] and usually reflect considerations such as avoidable morbidity and mortality, inappropriate variation in performance, and health service expenditure. Such criteria then inform questions such as: 'Is there a problem in healthcare provision or in health outcomes (informed by the availability of audit data) and are there guidelines that cover this problem?'

The nature of the healthcare organisation

When introducing clinical practice guidelines to improve patient care a number of characteristics of the organisation will be important. At the simplest level the size and complexity of the organisation will affect the feasibility of different strategies. Strategies for a primary care trust or a single general practice may well be inappropriate in an acute or mental health trust. For example, a strategy that involves face-to-face contact between a guidelines facilitator and all clinicians may be realistic for general practices but more difficult, if not impossible, within a large trust.

The culture of an organisation, specifically its approach and response to change, will also affect how guideline introduction should be approached. An organisation that has the ability to adapt to frequent change will offer different barriers and facilitators from one that is orientated towards maintaining the *status quo*. A key factor in an organisation's capacity to change and to implement guidelines is clinical leadership.[6,7]

Resources

The introduction of clinical practice guidelines requires resources. These include the costs of guidelines production but these are dwarfed by the time of appropriately skilled and experienced individuals who will conduct dissemination and implementation. At an organisational level the following skills are needed: knowledge of the theoretical basis of healthcare professional behaviour change and the empirical evidence about the effectiveness of different dissemination and implementation strategies; good interpersonal skills; knowledge of guideline development and appraisal methods. There may also be a need for specific skills for monitoring guidelines use: data processing skills for audit and feedback data or data collection skills for non-routine clinical data.

Finally, the introduction of guidelines will require the resources of clinicians within the organisation to participate in prioritisation and guideline adaptation (*see* below) and also to use clinical practice guidelines in the care of patients. Ideally, the healthcare organisation needs to make a corporate decision to commit these resources and protect the time of individuals involved.

Finding valid guidelines to use

Most healthcare organisations do not have adequate resources and skills to develop valid guidelines *de novo*.[4,8] Instead, we recommend that healthcare organisations should attempt to identify previously developed rigorous guidelines and adapt these for local use.[8]

Identifying published guidelines

Identifying published clinical practice guidelines is problematic. Many guidelines are published in the grey literature and are not indexed in the commonly available bibliographic databases. A number of sources, including sites on the Internet, catalogue clinical practice guidelines (Box 5.1). It is likely that such sites will become the best source to identify guidelines in the future with an increasing number giving full text versions or detailed abstracts of guidelines. In England and Wales, the National Institute for Clinical Excellence (www.nice.org.uk) has an ambitious guideline development programme, including a substantial portfolio of mental health guidelines. The first, on the management of schizophrenia, is being followed by nine more over the next three years. These guidelines have been developed with rigorous methods and reviewed by professional and lay stakeholders, as are those from SIGN, the Scottish Intercollegiate Guidelines Network[9] (www.sign.ac.uk), the first national guidelines programme in Europe.

If organisations cannot find published valid guidelines relevant to their identified priorities they face the choice of either amending their priorities or seeking to develop a guideline *de novo*. If they decide to develop a guideline, they should use as rigorous a method as possible within the resources available[4] and be explicit about the development methods and their potential limitations. The increasing availability of high-quality systematic reviews in the Cochrane Database of Systematic Reviews and the Cochrane Controlled Trial Register (both available in the Cochrane Library: www.update-software.com/clibng/cliblogon.htm[10]) make this task slightly less daunting than previously.

Appraising guidelines

There are potential biases inherent in guideline development that need to be addressed to maximise the validity of the resulting guideline. When an organisation has identified relevant guidelines, it is important to appraise their validity before deciding whether to adopt their recommendations.[11]

Box 5.1: Identifying guidelines

Search terms for common bibliographic databases
- MEDLINE and Healthstar – *guideline* (publication type) and *consensus development conference* (publication type) (Note: Healthstar includes non-MEDLINE-referenced journals and grey literature, e.g. government agency guidelines)
- CINAHL – *practice guidelines* (publication type) (Note: includes full text version of some guidelines)
- EMBASE - *practice guidelines* (subject heading) (Note: this is used for both articles about, and which contain, practice guidelines; furthermore the term was only introduced in 1994)

Useful websites
- National Institute for Clinical Excellence (NICE) – www.nice.org.uk/nice-web
- Scottish Intercollegiate Guidelines Network (SIGN) – full text versions of guidelines and quick reference guides (pc47.cee.hw.ac.uk/sign/home.htm)
- US National Guidelines Clearing House – www.guideline. gov
- Canadian Medical Association Clinical Practice Guidelines Infobase – index of clinical practice guidelines includes downloadable full text versions or abstracts for most guidelines (www.cma.ca/cpgs/index.html)
- German Guideline Clearing House – www.leitlinien.de/ggc.htm

---

If organisations adopt recommendations from guidelines of questionable validity, this may lead to harm to patients or wasteful use of resources on ineffective interventions. Guidelines from SIGN and NICE are thoroughly appraised before publication. If appraised guidelines are not available, organisations should undertake their own appraisal. The gold standard for the appraisal of guidelines, focusing on development methods, is the AGREE instrument (www.agreecollaboration.org). We suggest that healthcare organisations should only consider guidelines that report development methods explicitly by including a methods section within the guideline or supporting papers.[12,13] Without such information it is impossible to appraise the validity of guidelines and, as a result, difficult to have confidence in a guideline's recommendations.

Adaptation of valid guidelines

Once a group has identified guidelines of acceptable quality, they need to be adapted for use within the local healthcare setting. The first step is to set up a multidisciplinary group. Since for most clinical conditions good healthcare is dependent upon a multidisciplinary team, guideline implementation should be planned from this perspective. In terms of composition and function, this group will parallel the original guideline development group[4] but will not need systematic reviewing and evidence-summarising skills. The task of the group is to adapt the guideline and then plan the presentation, use and evaluation of the guideline within the local setting. Adaptation of the guideline involves reformatting the guideline recommendations in terms of measurable criteria and targets for quality improvement.[3] This is particularly necessary given the general nature of most guidelines.

Two main factors will influence how a guideline is adapted by a local group: the strength of recommendation within the guidelines, and local circumstances. As a result of the subjective element involved in the interpretation of evidence when deriving recommendations, there is always the potential for a group to reinterpret evidence and derive different recommendations. Deciding whether or not to derive different recommendations should be based, in large part, on the nature of the supporting evidence. Local adaptation groups should be wary of changing recommendations based upon good evidence but may want to change recommendations based upon weak evidence. Where recommendations based on good evidence are changed, the reasons for this should be explicitly stated.

In thinking about the use of the guideline, the group will take account of specific local circumstances. The North of England Evidence-Based Guideline on the use of ACE inhibitors in the management of patients with heart failure[14] suggests that, owing to the poor precision of clinical diagnosis, the diagnosis should be confirmed by echocardiography. The local adaptation of this recommendation will be influenced by whether open access facilities are available or whether access to echocardiography is via a cardiologist. A guideline adaptation group will then need to consider presentation, delivery, use and evaluation of the guideline as part of a coherent strategy.

Presentation
There will be a range of presentations from the full version of the guideline, summary sheets of all or part of the guideline, reminder sheets in patient records or various prompts such as guideline-related logos on mugs, pens or post-it pads. These strategies will overlap with use of the guideline when reminder sheets or computer templates are embedded within the patient record[15] or when test ordering forms are redesigned to encourage the gathering of appropriate clinical data. The role of guidelines integrated into electronic record systems is still not clear. In one recent trial computerised guidelines for the management of asthma and angina in general practice did not improve the quality of care,[16] yet it

is difficult to say there is no role for computerised guidelines in the world of electronic medical records.

Dissemination and implementation

Since there is no single effective way to ensure the use of guidelines in practice,[17–19] organisations should use multifaceted interventions to disseminate and implement guidelines. The choice of strategies should be informed by available resources, perceived barriers to care and research evidence about the effectiveness and efficiency of different strategies.[20] Systematic reviews of rigorous evaluations of dissemination and implementation strategies will provide the best evidence about their effectiveness and efficiency. Fortunately, there are an increasing number of systematic reviews of such strategies; in particular, the Cochrane Effective Practice and Organisation of Care Group[21] undertakes systematic reviews of interventions designed to improve quality of care, including professional interventions (e.g. continuing medical education, audit and feedback, reminders), organisational interventions (e.g. the expanded role of pharmacists), financial interventions (e.g. professional incentives) and regulatory interventions.

There are a variety of potential professional and organisational strategies that address different barriers. For example, educational approaches (attendance at seminars and workshops) may be useful where barriers relate to healthcare professionals' knowledge. Audit and feedback may be useful when healthcare professionals are unaware of suboptimal practice. Social influence approaches (local consensus processes, educational outreach, opinion leaders, marketing, etc.) may be useful when barriers relate to the existing culture, routines and practices of healthcare professionals. Reminders and patient-mediated interventions may be useful when healthcare professionals have problems processing information within consultations. Information about existing barriers can be collected by interviews with individual patients or clinicians, group interviews or direct observation. The presence of organisational barriers may require specific interventions. For example, in east London, the development of primary care dyspepsia guidelines led to the commissioning of a direct-access *Helicobacter pylori* testing service for general practitioners.

Evaluation

Evaluation is important to ensure that the process of care reflects guideline recommendations. The necessary data to allow this should be specified at the outset and should be linked to areas of strong evidence within the guideline.[22] Reminders or prompt sheets can be designed to encourage the recording of specific data items.[17,23]

Mental health or acute trust audit or clinical governance departments have a key role to play in collecting, analysing and feeding back these data. Clinical governance will depend on accurate and meaningful data about quality of care. We believe that criteria for clinical governance should be derived, at least in part, from the recommendations framed in evidence-based clinical practice guidelines.

Using guidelines for individual healthcare professionals

Outside a formal structure for the implementation of clinical practice guidelines within an organisation, individual clinicians may use guidelines as an information source for continuing professional education. Valid clinical practice guidelines provide an overview of the management of a condition or the use of an intervention. In this context, we argue that guidelines have potential advantages over systematic reviews. Guidelines usually have a broader scope than systematic reviews, which tend to focus on an individual problem or intervention. They may also provide a more coherent integrated view on how to manage a condition. Guidelines can also be used as instruments for self-assessment or peer review to learn about gaps in performance. Use of guidelines could become part of appraisal and revalidation. This is particularly relevant when the recommendations have been turned into specific measurable criteria.

Clinicians may also use guidelines to answer specific clinical questions arising out of their day-to-day practice. A key step is to frame the clinical question of interest in such a way that it can be answered specifying the patient or problem, the intervention of interest and possible comparison interventions and the outcomes of interest (see Sackett *et al.*[24] for a further discussion of this). This allows the clinician to identify what sort of evidence to search for. Under these circumstances clinical practice guidelines are only one of many types of evidence that are potentially relevant (systematic reviews, individual trials, expert advice).

Conclusions

Clinical practice guidelines are a part of current practice and will become increasingly common over the next decade. In this book we have suggested that great care needs to be taken both to maximise the validity of guidelines and ensure use within clinical practice. The latter requires adaptation for a local setting, good clinical leadership and the imaginative use of implementation strategies, preferably based on research evidence, tailored to relevant local factors. However, the implementation of clinical practice guidelines is not a panacea for improving clinical practice. They are one of a number of potential strategies that can help improve the quality of care that patients receive.[25]

References

1   Lomas J (1994) Teaching old (and not so old) docs new tricks: effective ways to implement research findings. In: EV Dunn, PG Norton, M Stewart *et al.* (eds) *Disseminating Research/Changing Practice. Research methods for primary care, Vol. 6.* Sage Publications, Thousand Oaks, CA.

2   Griffiths C and Feder G (1998) Using clinical guidelines in a general practitioner consultation. In: L Risdale (ed.) *Evidence-based Practice in Primary Health Care.* Churchill Livingstone, London.

3   Grimshaw J and Eccles M (1998) Clinical practice guidelines. In: C Silagy and A Haines (eds) *Evidence Based Practice in Primary Care.* BMJ Books, London.

4   Shekelle PG, Woolf SH, Eccles M *et al.* (1998) *Clinical Guidelines: developing guidelines.* BMJ Books, London.

5   NHS Executive (1996) *Clinical Guidelines: using clinical guidelines to improve patient care within the NHS.* NHSE, Leeds.

6   Ham C (2003) Improving the performance of health services: the role of clinical leadership. *Lancet.* **361:** 1978–80.

7   Bradley EH, Holmboe ES, Mattera JA *et al.* (2001) A qualitative study of increasing beta-blocker use after myocardial infarction: why do some hospitals succeed? *J Am Med Assoc.* **285:** 2604–11.

8   Royal College of General Practitioners (1996) *The Development and Implementation of Clinical Guidelines: Report of the Clinical Guidelines Working Group. Report from Practice, 26.* RCGP, Exeter.

9   Petrie JC, Grimshaw JM and Bryson A (1995) The Scottish Intercollegiate Guidelines Network initiative: getting validated guidelines into local practice. *Health Bull.* **53:** 345–8.

10 Cochrane Collaboration (1998) *The Cochrane Library* (3e). BMJ Publishing Library, London.

11 Cluzeau F, Littlejohns P and Grimshaw JM (1994) Appraising clinical guidelines – towards a 'Which' guide for purchasers. *Qual Health Care.* **3:** 121–2.

12 Eccles MP, Clapp Z, Grimshaw JM *et al.* (1996) North of England evidence based guidelines development project: methods of guideline development. *BMJ.* **312:** 760–1.

13 Eccles M, Freemantle N and Mason J (1998) Methods of developing guidelines for efficient drug use in primary care: North of England evidence based guidelines development project. *BMJ.* **316:** 1232–5.

14 Eccles M, Freemantle N and Mason J for the North of England ACE-inhibitor Guideline Development Group (1998) North of England evidence-based guideline development project: evidence-based guideline for the use of ACE-inhibitors in the primary care management of adults with symptomatic heart failure. *BMJ.* **316:** 1369–75.

15 Feder G, Griffiths C, Highton C *et al.* (1995) Do clinical guidelines introduced with practice based education improve care of asthmatic and diabetic patients? A randomised controlled trial in general practices in east London. *BMJ.* **311:** 1473–8.

16 Eccles M, McColl E, Steen N *et al.* (2002) Effect of computerised evidence based guidelines on management of asthma and angina in adults in primary care: cluster randomised controlled trial. *BMJ.* **325:** 941.

17 Effective Health Care (1994) *Implementing Clinical Practice Guidelines*. Bulletin No. 8. University of Leeds, Leeds.

18 Oxman AD, Thomson MA, Davis DA *et al.* (1995) No magic bullets: a systematic review of 102 trials of interventions to improve professional practice. *Can Med Assoc J.* **153**: 1423–31.

19 Wensing M and Grol R (1994) Single and combined strategies for implementing changes in primary care: a literature review. *Int J Qual Health Care.* **6**: 115–32.

20 Grol R (1997) Beliefs and evidence in changing clinical practice. *BMJ.* **315**: 418–21.

21 Bero L, Grilli R, Grimshaw JM *et al.* (eds) (1998) *The Cochrane Effective Practice and Organisation of Care Review Group. The Cochrane Database of Systematic Reviews* (2e). BMJ Books, London.

22 Agency for Health Care Policy and Research (1995) *Using Clinical Guidelines to Evaluate Quality of Care, Vol. 1: Issues*. US Department of Health and Human Services, Rockville, MD.

23 Emslie C, Grimshaw J and Templeton A (1993) Do clinical guidelines improve general practice management and referral of infertile couples? *BMJ.* **306**: 1728–31.

24 Sackett DL, Richardson WS, Rosenberg W *et al.* (1996) *Evidence Based Medicine. How to practice and teach EBM.* Churchill Livingstone, London.

25 Campbell SM, Steiner A, Robison J *et al.* (2003) Is the quality of care in general medical practice improving? Results of a longitudinal observational study. *Br J Gen Pract.* **53**: 298–304.

Chapter 6

The Mental Health Technology Appraisal and Clinical Guidelines Programmes of the National Institute for Clinical Excellence for England and Wales

Peter Littlejohns, Gillian Leng and Carole Longson

The National Institute for Clinical Excellence (NICE) was established in 1999 to provide national guidance on the clinical and cost-effectiveness of treatments and care for people using the NHS in England and Wales.

Mental health is one of the government's priority areas and a range of guidance products have been developed by the Institute to support implementation of the National Service Framework for Mental Health in England and its equivalent in Wales. In its first four years the Institute has issued guidance on six (out of a total of 60) technology appraisals and two newly commissioned guidelines (out of a total of three) that are related to the general area of mental health. Another seven relevant guidelines and two relevant appraisals are in preparation (*see* Chapter 8). The transparent and inclusive approach that the Institute has adopted in reaching its decisions has highlighted difficult technical and social issues facing the NHS as it seeks to balance its responsibility for enhancing services for individuals as well as improving the overall public health.

This chapter describes the processes of appraising technologies and developing guidelines and addresses some of the issues of integrating differing levels of guidance.

The role of the Institute

The National Institute for Clinical Excellence (NICE) was established as a special Health Authority in April 1999. It has four main aims.

1 To speed up the uptake by the National Health Service (NHS) of interventions that are both clinically and cost-effective.
2 To encourage more equitable access to healthcare (i.e. 'reduce post-code variation in care').

3 To provide better and more rational use of available resources by focusing the provision of healthcare on the most cost-effective interventions.

4 To encourage the creation of new and innovative technologies.

The Institute achieves these aims by providing guidance to the NHS in England and Wales on the effectiveness and cost-effectiveness of clinical interventions. This task is achieved by appraising new and existing technologies, developing disease-specific clinical guidelines and initially by supporting clinical audit (although the responsibility for the latter has transferred to the newly established Commission for Health Audit and Inspection, CHAI). In addition, the Institute has responsibility for the seven national confidential enquiries (including The Confidential Enquiry into Suicide and Homicide in People with a Mental Disorder), and more recently for assessing the safety and efficacy of new interventional procedures (previously the responsibility of SERNIP – Safety and Efficacy Register of New Interventional Procedures) and advising on the safety of borderline substances.

Quality improvement

The Institute's position in the broader quality improvement picture is illustrated in Figure 6.1. Its establishment has been part of the government's

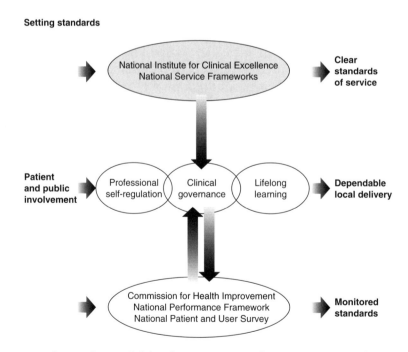

Figure 6.1: The quality model for the NHS. National Service Frameworks will set out common standards across the country for the treatment of particular conditions. NICE will act as a nationwide appraisal body for new and existing treatments and disseminate consistent advice on what works and what does not. *Source: A First Class Service: quality in the new NHS.*[2]

approach to improving the quality of the NHS outlined in the White Papers entitled *The New NHS: modern, dependable*[1] and *A First Class Service: quality in the new NHS*.[2] Standards for service configuration are established at a national level through the creation of national service frameworks, and clinical standards are established through the guidance issued by NICE.

The approach was initially presented as a 'quality improvement' model, with education and support being the key driving forces. However, a reduction in public and professional confidence in some of the systems currently in place to assure professional standards and institutional performance has resulted in tough messages from government. Politicians have sought to replace an 'educational' model with a more directive 'performance management' approach.

In this context, the Institute considers that one of its main roles is to provide guidance on controversial health issues where lack of clarity has resulted in regional variation in the care provided by the NHS. The guidance is considered to be a 'national standard' for clinical practice and is expected to be incorporated into local clinical governance mechanisms via the use of local guidelines and protocols. Monitoring of its uptake forms part of the assessment of local trusts undertaken by CHAI.

The Institute is a special Health Authority governed by a board consisting of executive and non-executive members, which meets in public (around the country) every two months. It is a small organisation (around 90 employees) based in London and undertakes its work by commissioning and liaising with a range of professional, specialist and patient organisations. It is supported by a Partner's Council, which includes representatives from all its stakeholders (including the pharmaceutical and medical devices industries). There are formal links with a number of universities and the NHS Research and Development (R&D) programme. The Institute works closely with local trusts and clinical governance professionals to ensure support for those responsible for implementing its guidance. This includes providing audit advice to accompany its guidance.

Evidence-based healthcare policy

The initial step in all technology appraisals and guideline development is to systematically search the literature for research evidence and estimate the magnitude of effect of the relevant interventions (for both costs and benefits) by statistical and modelling techniques. In practice the data required for the assessment of clinical and cost-effectiveness are usually deficient. This is because the research base necessary to assess clinical and cost-effectiveness is more extensive than that required for the initial licensing of a technology based solely on efficacy and safety. Many drugs for the treatment of mental health problems have been licensed on the basis of short-term trials which makes assessing the impact on chronic disease difficult.

The Institute recognises the important difference between 'assessment' of the research evidence and 'appraisal', which represents the translation of *all* the available evidence (including patient and professional experience) into practical guidance that is useful to the NHS on a day-to-day basis. Thus, while the guidance produced is firmly based on published evidence, it is also significantly influenced by the submissions from a variety of stakeholders, including professional organisations, patient/carer groups and the industry. It is apparent that results from the same evidence base can be interpreted differently, depending on the value given to different outcomes by each stakeholder. The final guidance issued by the Institute always draws upon the value judgements inherent to each stakeholder group. This is why it is essential to involve all these groups in the process. The Institute as part of its own research and development strategy has initiated a number of projects seeking to understand more fully how to integrate information from various sources into its decision-making processes; for example, the Patient Impact Assessment Feasibility project undertaken by Birmingham University and the value that the public place on a QALY undertaken in conjunction with the methodological section of the NHS R&D programme (www.publichealth.bham.ac.uk/nccrm/publications.htm).

Despite the volume and robustness of the evidence base for an intervention, judgement is always necessary when translating clinical research findings into guidance and can stimulate considerable controversy when the results determine national policy. An American sociologist, David Mechanic, argues that 'Research is a form of currency, as varying interests negotiate a political solution, but research is never definitive to resolve major issues on which strong political interests differ'.[3]

The stakes are now very high as the acceptance of a new intervention can have an enormous financial as well as a therapeutic impact. Even clinical research laboratories involved in developing innovative treatments can expect financial reward for contributing to a successful market drug.

In summary, although the Institute's approach to decision making is evidence based, pure research evidence is necessary but it is not sufficient alone. Additionally, in order that the decisions made are robust and credible the process has to be transparent, consultative, inclusive of all key stakeholders and responsive to change. These principles underpin all of the guidance issued by the Institute.

Enacting NICE principles in technology appraisals

When a technology appraisal is referred to the Institute from the Department of Health and the National Assembly for Wales, all possible stakeholders are identified. They are then consulted on the scope of the appraisal. An independent review of the published literature is commissioned from a university department through the NHS R&D programme.

In addition, the Institute receives submissions (both written and verbal) from all the stakeholders. The independent multidisciplinary appraisal committee considers all this information and consults on its provisional views (appraisal consultation document) via the Institute's website. The appraisal committee reconsiders its initial decision in the light of the comments and produces a final appraisal determination, which is placed on the website. Stakeholders can appeal against it if they consider the Institute and the guidance have not fulfilled a number of criteria. The Institute then issues the guidance to the NHS. A full description of the process and the principles underlying the appraisal decision-making process is available on www.nice.org.uk. Appraisals relevant to mental health issued so far include:

- newer atypical antipsychotic drugs for schizophrenia
  www.nice.org.uk/Docref.asp?d=32922
- computerised cognitive behavioural therapy for anxiety and depression
  www.nice.org.uk/Docref.asp?d=38248
- donepezil, rivastigmine and galantamine for Alzheimer's disease
  www.nice.org.uk/Docref.asp?d=14412
- methylphenidate for attention deficit disorder
  www.nice.org.uk/Docref.asp?d=11653
- electroconvulsive therapy
  www.nice.org.uk/Docref.asp?d=68306
- new drugs for bipolar disorders
  www.nice.org.uk/Docref.asp?d=86783

Enacting NICE principles in clinical practice guideline development

NICE produces clinical practice guidelines for the NHS in England and Wales in response to a referral from the Department of Health and the Welsh Assembly. The resultant work programme is now one of the most extensive programmes of guideline development in the world, with the capacity to have over 30 guidelines under production at any one time. It is based on internationally agreed standards for guideline development,[4] including evaluation of the best available evidence of clinical and cost-effectiveness, and an extensive stakeholder consultation process.

NICE guidelines in mental health

There are currently a large number of guideline topics relevant to mental health on the NICE work programme and it is anticipated that these will eventually span the whole breadth of the mental health field. Current topics that are either published or under development are listed in Chapter 8 and details of the publication status of these guidelines can be found on the NICE website (www.nice.org.uk).

Links with National Service Frameworks

The focus of a clinical practice guideline is to provide recommendations for healthcare professionals on the appropriate management of people with specific diseases or conditions. This is in contrast to a National Service Framework (NSF) where recommendations emphasise service delivery rather than individual patient care. The two programmes should be complementary, with NICE guidelines providing recommendations on best practice in clinical management, supported by recommendations in the NSFs describing how services should be configured to enable health-care professionals to deliver this best practice. Regular communication between teams developing guidelines and NSFs is therefore essential to ensure the boundaries between the work are clear and any overlapping issues are discussed. Detail on the links between NICE guidelines and the NSF for Mental Health are given in Chapter 8.

Integration of appraisals and guidelines

The appraisal programme was established to assess the correct positioning of a single intervention in the management of a disease on the basis of its clinical and cost-effectiveness. A guideline in the same clinical area addresses the broader context in which the single intervention fits. This differentiation ensures that a single intervention (usually but not always a drug) does not dominate the guideline developers' time at the expense of other therapeutic interventions. It also ensures that the sponsor of the technology can be assured that the Institute has given due consideration to all aspects of assessing its value.

It is apparent that with two guidance development processes advising the Institute on a similar clinical issue, there needs to be good integration of the development systems. This is achieved by close liaison between appraisal and guideline technical staff within the Institute, attendance of the guideline development group chairman at the appraisal meetings, and consultee status of the guideline development group for any relevant appraisal. In the end there has to be clarity over the roles of each development process and the Institute's policy is that the guideline development group is required to adopt the recommendations of the appraisal process when appropriate into the guideline.

The first full mental health guideline issued by the Institute was on the management of schizophrenia and this incorporated the appraisal on the use of newer atypical antipsychotics.

National Collaborating Centres

NICE commissions seven National Collaborating Centres (NCCs) to develop the guidelines on its work programme. Each Centre is a

multidisciplinary collaboration of healthcare professionals, user representatives and technical experts. The Centres have the capacity, skills and
expertise to deliver guidelines that are of a high quality, each with the
following attributes:

- led by professionals with requisite academic support
- work closely with patient and carer representatives
- complement each other, sharing skills and expertise co-operatively
- have governance arrangements that assure co-operation, wide participation, consultation and clear contractual accountability.

The Centres are largely based in medical royal colleges and cover a range
of clinical areas (Table 6.1). Further details on the Centre for Mental
Health are given in Chapter 8.

Table 6.1: National Collaborating Centres and their host organisations.

National Collaborating Centre	Host organisation
Acute Care	Royal College of Surgeons
Cancer	Velindre NHS Trust, Wales
Chronic Conditions	Royal College of Physicians
Nursing and Supportive Care	Royal College of Nursing
Mental Health	British Psychological Society
	Royal College of Psychiatrists
Primary Care	Royal College of General Practitioners
Women's and Children's Health	Royal College of Obstetricians and Gynaecologists

The guideline development process

The development of NICE clinical practice guidelines is a joint process
shared between the NCCs and the Institute, with input at several stages
from relevant stakeholders. Stakeholders are those organisations with an
interest in the guideline topic, including national patient or professional
bodies, companies manufacturing relevant drugs or medical devices, and
NHS organisations. Stakeholder input is vital to ensure all aspects have
been appropriately addressed in the guideline and to support implementation. Guideline development is therefore a complex process, taking on
average two years to complete each guideline.

The process of guideline development can be divided into four phases as
described in Table 6.2. More details on each of the phases are given in the
guideline manuals available on the NICE website (www.nice.org.uk), and
specifically in relation to the development of mental health guidelines in
Chapter 8.

Table 6.2:   Phases in NICE guideline development.

Development phase	Key components
1 Initiation	• Topic referred to NICE by the Department of Health and the Welsh Assembly • NICE commissions appropriate NCC to develop guideline • Stakeholders register interest • NCC develops scope outlining areas to be covered within the guideline for consultation with stakeholders • NCC agrees methodology for guideline development with NICE

2 Development	• NCC convenes a multidisciplinary guideline development group, including patients and carers to:
	  – define key clinical questions relevant to the topic area
	  – review best evidence of clinical and cost-effectiveness, including stakeholder submissions
	  – produce recommendations and write the guideline for submission to NICE
	• NICE provides technical input as required

3 Validation and publication	• NICE sends guideline to stakeholders for two four-week periods of consultation • NCC revises guideline to take into account stakeholder views as appropriate • NICE approves final guideline in conjunction with the guideline review panel (*see* below) • NICE and NCC publish and disseminate the guideline • Implementation of guideline supported by the NCC and NICE as appropriate
4 Review and update	NCC updates the guideline between two and four years after publication, depending on whether significant new evidence is available

Guideline review panels

Seven guideline review panels have been established to advise and assist in the guideline work programme. Each panel is aligned to one NCC. The panel members provide external validation for the guidelines by overseeing the development process, advising on the commissioning of work and monitoring the quality of the guidelines. Members are expected to have an in-depth knowledge of the development of their allocated guidelines and keep a record of the documents relating to their guidelines.

Publication

Guidelines commissioned by NICE are published in three formats, making it easier for different groups to access the information most relevant to them.

The NICE guideline

This is a short summary publication containing all the recommendations produced by the guideline development group. A small number of recommendations are prioritised by the group as 'key' recommendations, representing those considered to have the greatest impact on patient care, and these are suggested as priorities for implementation. The NICE guideline also contains additional information on implementation, to advise local NHS bodies on how to approach the guideline and to make them aware of any other relevant national initiatives such as NSFs.

Information for the public

This publication mirrors the NICE guideline, presenting guideline recommendations in lay language to make them more widely accessible. It also provides some background information about the condition covered by the guideline to help put the recommendations in context.

The full guideline

This contains all the guideline recommendations, but also includes much more detailed information for interested specialists in the field. It includes detail on the development process, a description of how the evidence was collected, reviewed and assessed, plus full reference details of the relevant literature, detail on how the recommendations were formulated and recommendations for future research.

Implementation

Successful implementation is key to the success of the guideline programme. NICE and the NCCs are both involved in dissemination of the guidelines and help to support implementation through professional organisations and patient groups. Wherever possible, NICE encourages other organisations to republish the recommendations in the most appropriate format to support local use, for example through the development of protocols.

Conclusions

NICE has been given an ambitious work programme. It issues guidance to the NHS in various formats, each with its own development process and yet all adhering to the Institute's core principles. Its activities are likely to increase with the Institute's imminent involvement in advising on national screening programmes.

The challenge in the future will be to ensure that all these programmes are fully integrated. It is imperative that an individual patient, professional or member of the public interested in a particular disease can be assured that there are national evidence-based standards of clinical practice that cover all aspects of care from prevention through to palliation.

References

1 Department of Health (1997) *The New NHS: modern, dependable*. HMSO, London.
2 Department of Health (1998) *A First Class Service: quality in the new NHS*. HMSO, London.
3 Mechanic D (1993) Social research in health and the American sociopolitical context: the changing fortunes of medical sociology. *Soc Sci Med*. 36: 95–102.
4 Cluzeau FA, Burgers JS, Brouwers M *et al.* (2003) Development and validation of an international appraisal instrument for assessing the quality of clinical practice guidelines: the AGREE project. *Qual Safety Health Care*. 12(1): 18–23.

Chapter 7

Mental health guidelines development in Scotland

Joanne Topalian and Sara Twaddle

A 1990 report by the Scottish Executive's Clinical Resource and Audit Group highlighted the need for national, evidence-based clinical guidelines to be developed by 'the Royal Colleges, the specialist associations of the healthcare professionals and relevant educational bodies'.[1] As a result of this, and the personal enthusiasm and determination of the late Professor James Petrie, the Scottish Intercollegiate Guidelines Network (SIGN) was established in 1993 by the Conference of Royal Colleges and their faculties in Scotland, to develop evidence-based clinical guidelines for the National Health Service in Scotland.[2]

Since 1993 SIGN has published 75 guidelines and has become a world-leading organisation in the development of evidence-based guidelines. Multiprofessional involvement at all stages of the guideline development process has been a fundamental principle of SIGN methodology since it began, though the extent of such involvement has increased in recent years. SIGN Council, the major decision-making body for SIGN, now has representation from all medical Royal Colleges and faculties, patient organisations, organisations representing nursing, midwifery, pharmacy, allied health professions, social work and health service management. The National Health Service in Scotland funds SIGN, through a grant from NHS Quality Improvement Scotland (NHS QIS).

Each year SIGN produces between nine and 12 guidelines covering a range of conditions from day-case cataract surgery to hypertension in the elderly to epithelial ovarian cancer. All published guidelines can be viewed at www.sign.ac.uk.

The first mental health guideline developed by SIGN was *Interventions in the Management of Behavioural and Psychological Aspects of Dementia*, published in February 1998. This guideline is currently being reviewed. This was followed by *Psychosocial Interventions in the Management of Schizophrenia* in October 1998. Since then, *Attention Deficit and Hyperkinetic Disorders in Children and Young People*, *Postnatal Depression and Puerperal Psychosis* and *The Management of Harmful Drinking and Alcohol Dependency in Primary Care* have been published in 2001, 2002 and 2003 respectively. A guideline on *Bipolar Affective Disorder* is in development, due to be completed by 2006.

Developing guidelines the SIGN way

This section summarises the SIGN approach to developing evidence-based clinical practice guidelines and discusses issues associated with developing guidelines in the mental health area.

The process of developing evidence-based guidelines has evolved significantly over the last 10 years, incorporating grading systems, patient involvement and consideration of the economic consequences of recommendations. In February 2001 SIGN published *SIGN50: A Guideline Developer's Handbook*, which sets out the SIGN development process (www.sign.ac.uk/guidelines/fulltext/50/index.html).

Choosing topics

The SIGN process allows anyone to suggest a topic for consideration via the completion of a standard application form. In parallel, SIGN has six specialty subgroups (mental health and learning disabilities; cancer; general and cardiovascular medicine; surgery; women, children and dental; primary care) that use their clinical networks to compile a list of potential guideline topics needed by health professionals. For each proposal received, SIGN performs a scoping search of the literature to give an indication of the size of the evidence base upon which such a guideline could be based. A Guideline Programme Advisory Group of SIGN Council then sifts this initial list of proposals into a shorter list using a screening tool that employs a number of criteria, including clinical importance, size of the evidence base and known variation in practice. The final proposed programme is decided by SIGN Council at its autumn meeting, using a second screening device that covers issues of importance of the topic to healthcare professionals, patients and carers, and the likely ability to implement the guideline in Scotland. The final stage of topic selection is undertaken by NHS QIS, who seek independent advice from clinical leaders and then finally approve the programme.

Forming a group

In many cases the chair of the guideline development group is the person who first proposed the topic to SIGN, subject to approval by SIGN Council. When this is not the case, nominations are requested from members of SIGN Council. The chair of the guideline development group has a role in identifying all relevant clinical specialties plus two general practitioners and two patient representatives. SIGN Council thereafter nominates individuals from their own specialist area to sit on the group.

SIGN programme managers facilitate guideline development by the guideline development group. They co-chair the group meetings and the setting and meeting of key deadlines. Each group also includes a SIGN information specialist, who undertakes the systematic literature search. An example of the composition of a guideline development group is shown in Box 7.1.

Box 7.1:   Composition of the Postnatal Depression and Puerperal Psychosis Guideline Development Group

- Community psychiatric nurse
- Consultant in public health medicine
- General practitioner
- Health economist
- Health visitors × 3
- Midwives × 2
- Obstetricians × 2
- Patient representatives × 2
- Pharmacist
- Psychiatrists × 2
- Psychologist
- Researcher in child and adolescent psychiatry
- SIGN programme manager and information officer
- Social worker
- Voluntary agency representative

Group members are invited to attend training courses in critical appraisal, tailored for levels of previous knowledge, to prepare them for the task of reviewing clinical literature.

Identifying the questions to be addressed by the guideline

Two key factors affect the choice of questions to be addressed by the guideline development group. The first is the issue of scope, that is, whether the guideline will attempt to address the whole spectrum of the patient's journey or take a more limited focus. In the first case the guideline would seek to address issues including screening, prevention, detection, management and treatment and in the second, the guideline would focus on specific stages of that journey. The second factor is the results from an early search for issues identified as important to patients and carers, which are presented to the group at their first meeting. In the light of these two factors the group identifies the key questions on which the systematic literature review will be based.

Systematic review of the evidence and considered judgement

Information specialists within the SIGN team undertake a systematic search of the literature to identify relevant papers for members of the guideline development group to appraise critically. Once a search has been conducted, retrieved abstracts are sifted to identify only the papers of direct relevance to the question being addressed. Systematic reviews and meta-analyses are reviewed before randomised controlled trials, case control studies and observational studies.

Once the group has sifted the papers, the selected papers are ordered and at least two group members review each paper, using critical appraisal checklists provided by SIGN. The information from the checklists is incorporated into evidence tables, which are reviewed by the group. However, the process of forming recommendations does not rely on evidence alone; a significant component of the process is the 'considered judgement' of the group based on their clinical experience and the clinical context in which they work. Considered judgement may, for example, take account of different ways in which services are delivered in Scotland, the availability of resources and any important issues identified by the patient representatives. This process is documented to allow those reviewing the guideline to identify the reasons why recommendations do not always directly mirror the published evidence in every case.

The group then bases the guideline upon the considered judgement forms, with the programme manager and group chair working together to produce a first draft for presentation at the first stage of peer review.

Peer review

The first stage of peer review is a national open meeting, where the first draft of the guideline is discussed by a wide audience of healthcare professionals and patients from all over Scotland. At the same time the guideline is placed on the website for one month to allow others to comment. The aim of the national open meeting is to generate discussion around how the guideline group has interpreted the evidence, any gaps in the guideline and the applicability of the recommendations.

After the national open meeting the group addresses the issues raised and update literature searches are undertaken. A new version of the guideline is produced and sent to experts in the field for critical review and suggested revision. Peer review comments received at this stage are all logged and a group response must be made to each comment. A further version of the guideline, incorporating the relevant peer review comments, is then prepared for the editorial process.

Editorial process

The editorial process for SIGN guidelines is undertaken in house, with input from the Chairman of SIGN, the Director, the Programme Director and a small group drawn from SIGN Council. This process ensures that the guideline group has responded appropriately to the peer review comments and also covers both technical editing and a 'reality check' on the recommendations made.

Publishing and distribution

Once published, SIGN guidelines are sent to all NHS organisations in Scotland for local distribution to the relevant healthcare professionals. In addition, all SIGN guidelines are posted on the SIGN website (www.sign. ac.uk) to allow access for patients, the public and international healthcare professionals. Local implementation of SIGN guidelines remains a responsibility of the NHS, but SIGN is increasingly working with colleagues to support initiatives to raise awareness and use of the guidelines.

Issues in the development of evidence-based clinical guidelines in mental health

The remainder of this chapter discusses issues for SIGN in developing evidence-based guidelines in the field of mental health and identifies challenges for the future.

Only a small number of SIGN guidelines are in the field of mental health. The reasons for this appear to be two-fold. First, a relatively small number of mental health topics are proposed to SIGN, and second, the mental health guideline topics that are proposed face tough competition to get onto the SIGN programme from the other national priority areas for health in Scotland (cancer, coronary heart disease and child health). These issues are highlighted in Table 7.1, which shows both the quantities and

Table 7.1: Guideline proposals to SIGN, by clinical area 2001–3, successful proposals in brackets.

	Mental health	Coronary and cardiovascular	Child health	Cancer	Other	Total
2003	3 (2)	None	2 (2)*	3 (2)	10 (3)	17
2002	3 (0)	4 (4)	1 (1)	2 (1)	5 (2)	15
2001	3 (2)	2 (2)	2 (2)	4 (4)	6 (2)	17
Total	9 (4)	6 (6)	5 (5)	9 (7)	21 (7)	50 (29)

* One of these is also classified as mental health.

the types of guideline proposals made to SIGN in the last three years. The numbers in brackets are the successful proposals.

Mental health and child health received the lowest number of proposals, yet 100% of the child health proposals were successful while only 44% of mental health proposals submitted to SIGN were voted onto the SIGN programme. These figures are more striking when compared to the 100% of cardiovascular and 77% of cancer proposals that were voted onto the SIGN programme. The situation with regard to mental health proposals may be improving: in 2003, of the 17 proposals considered by SIGN Council, three were mental health guideline proposals, two of which were accepted onto the SIGN programme.

Clearly then, only a small number of proposals for mental health guidelines are successful when compared with the other national priority areas for health in Scotland. The question should also be asked as to why relatively few mental health topics are proposed to SIGN in the first place.

SIGN is in the business of producing evidence-based guidelines so a proposal to SIGN is unlikely to be accepted unless it can demonstrate a significant evidence base. The field of mental health appears to suffer from a lack of high-quality evidence. Perhaps potential guideline proposers are aware of this, and the relatively low level of proposals reflects this poor evidence base.

We have explored this perception of a lack of high-quality evidence in mental health by examining a range of recently published SIGN guidelines in more detail (Table 7.2). The Postnatal Depression and Puerperal Psychosis guideline contains only five recommendations that are graded B or above, whereas the other guidelines listed contain between nine and 52 recommendations graded B or above. Similarly, 58% of recommendations in the Postnatal Depression and Puerperal Psychosis guideline are at the level of good practice points (GPP). The percentage of good practice points in the other guidelines ranges from 12 to 37%. Despite the fact that the grade of recommendation relates to the strength of the

Table 7.2:   Grade of recommendation by guideline.

	A	B	C	D	GPP	Total
59 – Lower respiratory tract infection	2	8	4	3	10	27
60 – Postnatal depression and puerperal psychosis	1	4	9	7	30	53
61 – Postmenopausal bleeding	2	7	4	4	6	23
62 – Prophylaxis of venous thromboembolism	45	7	33	15	14	114
64 –Management of patients with stroke	4	20	3	18	25	70

evidence and not clinical importance, the grade is a good indicator of the size and type of evidence base available, a key factor that is taken into account when SIGN Council votes for each proposal.

It could also be that those people who may want and need a SIGN mental health guideline (psychiatrists, psychologists, community psychiatric nurses and community groups amongst others) may be unaware that they can propose a topic to SIGN, an organisation that has historically been seen as physician led. Finally there is always the possibility that potential proposers have little interest and/or faith in the role of guidelines or in SIGN guidelines in particular. Some of the issues explored by the National Collaborating Centre for Mental Health in Chapter 8 may be relevant here.

Successful proposals

Despite the problems with getting mental health guideline topics on to the SIGN programme, those that have been produced to date have been highly praised by NHS Scotland.[3]

In 2002 SIGN piloted its first clinical launch of a guideline with the Postnatal Depression and Puerperal Psychosis guideline. The event was heavily oversubscribed and was evaluated very highly. Other guideline launches have followed, notably the launch of the Management of Harmful Drinking and Alcohol Dependency in Primary Care guideline that attracted 545 delegates. SIGN also regularly monitors how many guidelines are downloaded from the SIGN website. Figures for the period between 1 June and 11 November 2003 show that both the Postnatal Depression and Puerperal Psychosis and the Management of Harmful Drinking and Alcohol Dependency in Primary Care guidelines were among the top 25 downloaded guidelines.

The future

SIGN may need to do further work to raise awareness amongst practitioners and the wider public of how proposals for mental health guidelines can be submitted. Progress is already being made in this area with the recent expansion of the Mental Health and Learning Disability Specialty subgroup to include a wider range of specialties and service user representation. It may also be time for SIGN to consider making a special case for mental health proposals at the yearly SIGN Council voting meeting. The evidence base for mental health guidelines may not be as strong as in other fields but the need for them is just as great.

References

1 Scottish Office (1993) *Clinical Resource and Audit Group. Clinical Guidelines: a report by a Working Group.* Scottish Office, Edinburgh.
2 Petrie JC, Grimshaw JM and Bryson A (1995) The Scottish Intercollegiate Guidelines Network Initiative: getting validated guidelines into local practice. *Health Bull (Edinburgh).* **53**: 345–8.
3 Clinical Resource and Audit Group Implementation Sub-group (2002) *Implementation of SIGN Guidelines in NHS Scotland.* NHS Scotland, Edinburgh.

Chapter 8

The National Collaborating Centre for Mental Health

Tim Kendall and Steve Pilling

This chapter introduces the National Collaborating Centre for Mental Health (NCCMH) and its work on national clinical practice guidelines. We highlight the process of guideline production within the NCCMH, focusing upon the potential problems, both conceptual and practical, encountered along the 'journey' of producing guidelines in mental health. Some of the issues we raise will be shared with many other groups producing clinical practice guidelines. Others will not.

In mental health the process of treatment begins with an assessment of a person's history and 'mental state', including past and present behaviour, mood, affect, thoughts and beliefs, perceptions and cognitive function. In gathering this clinical evidence, a practitioner also needs to know about the person's social context and support, home circumstances, employment and educational opportunities, past treatments and current treatment preferences, hopes and aspirations, both in terms of the person's life aims and in terms of how treatment might help them achieve those life goals. This is a complex and highly individual process leading to an equally individual treatment plan.

Mental health services are multidisciplinary (psychiatrists, psychologists, occupational therapists, nurses, social workers and others) and provide a range of interventions (pharmacological, physical, psychological and social/service-level interventions*). Much of the treatment and care provided, especially in secondary services, is delivered by teams as a 'package' or 'programme' of care, involving different treatment types. Not infrequently, such care will involve staff from the statutory and voluntary sectors, each providing care in a number of different settings, including primary, secondary and tertiary health services, social services, at home, in voluntary organisations and other community settings.

---

* The latter includes a variety of interventions, some social and intended to be directly therapeutic (e.g. therapeutic communities), and others organisational and intended to deliver care more effectively and closer to a service user's home (e.g. crisis resolution and home treatment teams or assertive outreach teams).

The individual nature of mental health problems and their treatment, and the range and diversity of professionals and agencies involved in a person's care, might suggest that evidence-based guidelines drawn from a narrow base of effective interventions could not properly address the complexity of the problem. Moreover, the questionable validity of some diagnostic categories such as depression[1] and the substantial placebo effects in the treatment of many mental health problems[2] might suggest that any claim to a proper evidence base for the treatment and care of any mental health problem is at best premature. Whilst we accept that psychological disorders are likely to elude precise definition, and that mental health and social care is an amalgam of specific interventions provided against a background of humanity and compassion, our view is that clinical practice guidelines can bring together the best evidence for treatment with the need for compassion and care.

The National Collaborating Centre for Mental Health

The NCCMH, one of seven NCCs (*see* Chapter 6), was established by the National Institute for Clinical Excellence (NICE) in April 2001 specifically, but not exclusively, to generate evidence-based guidelines in mental health. The NCCMH is a collaboration (led by the Royal College of Psychiatrists and the British Psychological Society) between the key national professional organisations involved in mental health and social care, three leading national service user and carer organisations, two academic organisations who provide technical support, and NICE. Each organisation has a representative on the NCCMH Reference Group – the body that provides a strategic overview of the NCCMH activities.

The NCCMH is run by two co-directors and currently has just under 20 staff, with the capacity to develop six guidelines at any one time. Guidelines allocated, currently under way or completed are:

- schizophrenia (completed December 2002)[3]
  www.nice.org.uk/Docref.asp?d=42460
- eating disorders (completed January 2004)
  www.nice.org.uk/Docref.asp?d=101245
- depression (due to be completed June 2004)
- self-harm (due to be completed July 2004)
- depression in children (due to be completed mid-2005)
- post-traumatic stress disorder (due to be completed early 2005)
- obsessive compulsive disorder (due to be completed mid 2005)
- bipolar affective disorder (due to be completed mid 2006)
- dementia (due to start April 2004).

The choice of topics for guidelines is made by the Department of Health (DoH). Once selected, NICE, the NCCMH, the DoH and registered stakeholders negotiate the 'scope' of the guideline. At this stage there is often a tension between the stakeholders wanting the scope to cover the widest range of service users and interventions, while the NCCMH often prefers a more limited scope, upon which future expanded guidelines can be built. This negotiation, a frequently lengthy process, is facilitated by a close working relationship between NICE and the NCCMH and has the real advantage of gaining wider ownership and acceptance of the limits of the scope.

The guideline development group

Just as the NCCMH Reference Group must reflect the range of professionals involved in mental health work so should each guideline development group (GDG). GDGs include a chair, often with expertise in the condition in question, clinical or academic experts, a range of relevant 'jobbing practitioners', at least two service users and one carer, a facilitator (one of the co-directors), along with technical and research support from NCCMH staff.

Selecting the chair of the GDG is central to the success of the guideline. The chair should have a good grasp of the condition but does not have to be a recognised expert. However, they do need a high level of interpersonal skills to be able to facilitate a potentially disparate group of people together over 18 months, while also keeping the work plan on course and meeting pre-agreed deadlines. They also need to be able to write proficiently, understand the guideline development process and evidence-based practice and, crucially, have the time to devote to this lengthy process.

Once identified, the chair, in conjunction with one of the NCCMH co-directors and with advice from the NCCMH Reference Group and others, selects the other GDG members to form a group that is knowledgeable, representative and dynamic. Perhaps most importantly, they must 'get on' well enough to approach group and individual business with mutual respect and to undertake the reviewing of evidence collectively. To assist in this regard, a division of roles often emerges between the chair and co-director with the chair focusing on the management of business both internal and external to the group (the group task) and the co-director focusing on the management of the dynamics of the group (the group process).[4]

Service users and carers

Service users and carers are recruited with the support of the NICE Patient Involvement Unit (PIU). They have equal status to all other guideline members and have a particular and important contribution to make. Often this is most keenly felt by the professional members of the group when they are forced to face issues such as: the limits of the treatments they have to offer, the consequences of experiencing compulsory treatment under the Mental Health Act or the real variation in practice faced by service users and carers. This serves to remind professionals of the purpose of the guideline. The willingness and openness with which many service users speak of their experience also help health professionals to adopt a more open and practical approach to reviewing the clinical evidence. They also play a vital role in the final stages of generating recommendations, injecting both humility and harsh reality into the work of the group.

Typically, service users on GDGs help by setting the scene at the initial training day that is held for each guideline. Their role here is to describe to the rest of the GDG their experience of the disorder and its treatment and care. Service users and carers also undertake training in guideline methodology along with the rest of the GDG. The service user and carer focus is maintained throughout by having a standing agenda item specifically devoted to service user and carer concerns for every GDG meeting. Within the NCCMH, service users are encouraged to play a key role in the editing process, working particularly closely with the chair on the introduction. It almost goes without saying that the public version of any guideline must have input from service users and carers.

The guideline development process

Following training, the GDG explores the scope and generates the clinical questions that will guide the search for evidence. For larger guidelines such as schizophrenia or depression, the questions are often grouped under topic headings (e.g. pharmacological, psychological or service-level interventions) for consideration by sub-groups of the GDG ('topic groups' – TGs), led by a member of the GDG with expertise in the area. For many guidelines, special advisers are recruited to support the work of the TGs or the GDG as a whole. However, in all cases the work of the TG is referred back to the full GDG for discussion and agreement. Group members, within the TGs or the full guideline development group, also help guide the literature searches, identify marker papers for checking the effectiveness of search strategies, quality assure studies and interrogate data through systematic review and meta-analysis supported by NCCMH staff.

A hierarchical, step-wise approach to evidence identification and extraction has been developed by the NCCMH (for an example see the full schizophrenia guideline[3,5]). For data derived from RCTs, where appropriate standard meta-analytic techniques are applied, results are presented to the TG and GDG for discussion, analysis and generating statements. Statements for Level I evidence are developed systematically using a simple algorithm, which rests upon statistical significance, clinical significance (defined by the GDG) and confidence intervals (*see* Figure 8.1).

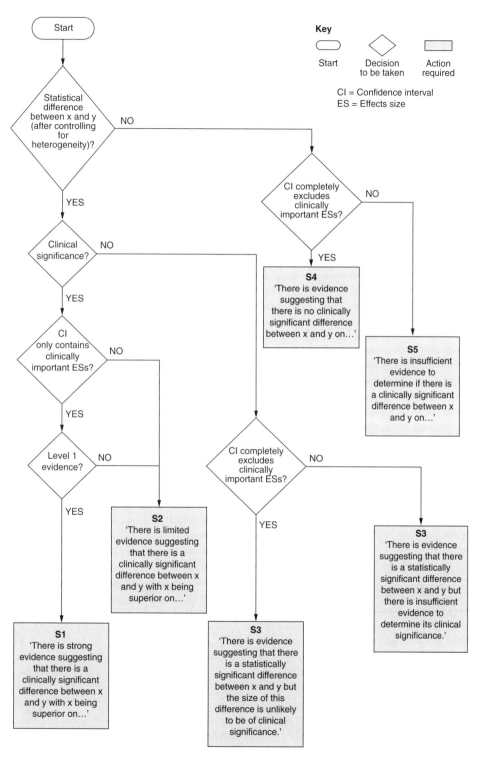

Figure 8.1: Guideline statement decision tree.

Currently the NCCMH does not employ formal consensus methods. Where appropriate RCT data for efficacy studies are unavailable, a descriptive or narrative review of identified best-quality research is undertaken, led by relevant GDG members supported by the NCCMH staff. This is an iterative process in which successive drafts are reviewed by TG members, NCCMH staff, specialist advisors and the wider GDG. On occasions, often where little or no high-quality evidence is available, national and international experts are invited to make presentations to the GDG, which can then guide the narrative review.

Health economic evidence

Good-quality health economic data are a rarity in mental health. Often little is known even about the basic healthcare costs associated with a particular disorder. Very few studies on cost-effectiveness have been published, and where they have, they are usually underpowered.

We have therefore usually taken two approaches to health economics: a cost-minimisation approach, and modelling of cost-effectiveness. For example, for the depression guideline, we used a cost-minimisation approach to compare various interventions, such as antidepressants, structured exercise and self-help, in the treatment of depression in primary care. In the eating disorder guideline, we developed a model to assess the cost-effectiveness for cognitive behavioural therapy (CBT) against antidepressants in the treatment of bulimia nervosa. This latter type of work is relatively resource intensive and so GDGs are encouraged to focus on one or two key questions per guideline. Whatever methods are used, an important challenge is enabling GDG members to understand the nature of health economic evidence: many struggle with health economic concepts and are often suspicious, assuming that health economics is simply about rationing or the exclusion of costly interventions from the NHS (*see also* Chapter 3).

Forming, grading and integrating recommendations

Moving from statements to recommendations is rarely straightforward for a number of reasons, some 'internal' to a guideline, some 'external'. External influences are primarily technical and include ensuring NICE technology appraisals and other NICE guidelines in mental health support rather than contradict recommendations in each new guideline produced by the NCCMH. With regard to the internal influences, two seem of particular relevance. They relate to service-level interventions (*see* above) and the make-up of trial populations and comparators, especially for trials undertaken in different healthcare systems. For example, in schizophrenia, studies of crisis resolution and home treatment teams (CRHTTs) have never evaluated the use of CRHTTs solely for people with schizophrenia, the population in trials reflecting a diagnostic mix of acute psychotic and non-psychotic disorders. Even though studies for inclusion were restricted to those in which the study population contained a majority of people with schizophrenia, recommendations for the use of CRHTTs for people with schizophrenia were necessarily extrapolated from the evidence for CRHTTs used for a more mixed clinical population, and to reflect this, recommendations were downgraded. Similarly, when reviewing the evidence for assertive outreach teams (AOTs) for people with schizophrenia, we found very good evidence for the superior effectiveness of AOTs over 'standard services' in the US, but exercised caution when developing recommendations for their use in the UK where 'standard services' are clearly different.

Consultation

The process of consultation described in Chapter 6 is crucial to the success and the acceptability of guidelines. The 200 pages of comments received for the schizophrenia guideline were a testament to the keen interest from all areas of mental health, including service user organisations, professional organisations, the pharmaceutical industry and the public.

   The comments often serve to highlight some of the tensions inherent in mental health guideline development. For example, GDGs have to reconcile the fact that service users and professionals are interested in different outcomes and place different emphases on the experience of care, the role of medication and access to 'talking therapies'. Moreover, most commentators – professional groups, consumer groups, the pharmaceutical industry – show a tendency towards self-interest in the comments and changes they suggest.

Dissemination and implementation

NICE's role is presently limited to the production and dissemination of guidance for the NHS. However, the NCCMH is moving to focus on implementation, exploiting the relationship to the relevant professional bodies. The NCCMH, with its base in the Royal College of Psychiatrists and the British Psychological Society and with wide support from other professional and service user/carer organisations within mental health, has direct connections with the professionals and service users and carers for whom the guidelines are intended. This can have an immediate impact; for example, the Royal College of Psychiatrists has already begun the process of modifying curricula for the training of psychiatrists in light of the schizophrenia guideline – a concrete example of the influence guidelines can have as a direct result of the placing, ownership and proximity of the NCCMH to its parent organisations.

For the schizophrenia guideline, the NCCMH produced a web-based (and CD-Rom version) 'training pack', freely available to anyone who can access the web (www.rcpsych.ac.uk/cru/sts/index.htm#). The National Institute of Mental Health in England (NIMHE, www.nimhe.org) funded the production and dissemination of the CD-Rom version. The NCCMH will work closely with NIMHE and its associated development centres in supporting the implementation of the schizophrenia and subsequent guidelines. An initial research programme within the NCCMH is also under way to examine barriers to guideline implementation in mental health services.

Specific problems for guidelines in mental health

We have identified some of the problems of guideline production and implementation, which are probably common to most clinical practice guidelines. For mental health, guidelines have a number of particular pitfalls and problems.

Diagnosis and diagnostic heterogeneity present problems for all types of quantitative research in mental health. Diagnostic criteria in mental health have been operationalised (ICD-10;[6] DSM-IV[7]), so improving the reliability of diagnoses. However, there has been little comparable improvement in the validity of diagnoses in mental health,[1] a situation resulting partly from our inability to confirm most diagnoses through physical tests and partly because current theories of aetiology and of the mechanisms of treatment are putative and lacking in specificity.

The result is that the larger diagnostic categories, such as depression, anxiety or schizophrenia, tend to be over-inclusive, reducing our ability to detect differences between competing treatments. For example, the manifest heterogeneity of people diagnosed with depression introduces substantial problems for finding evidence of benefit for specific treatments when evaluated for all people with the diagnosis. There is a clear need to evaluate specific treatments not by existing diagnostic groups but by yet to be defined diagnostic sub-groups or other patient characteristics. And for both psychological and pharmacological interventions, account should also be taken of the heterogeneity of professional characteristics, and how patient and professional characteristics interact.

Conversely, research focused on very tightly defined diagnostic categories, such as anorexia nervosa and bulimia nervosa, tend to be under-inclusive, most service users with eating disorders showing aspects of more than one diagnosis. Little research to date has addressed this demographically larger group of service users. A related issue in mental health is that of 'dual diagnosis'. For example, many people with the diagnosis of schizophrenia also have an alcohol or other substance misuse problem: little research has addressed the evidence base for the treatment of people with both diagnoses. Similar problems arise for guidelines for depression: a sizeable minority of people with this diagnosis also carry a diagnosis of personality disorder and there is little if any evidence for the treatment of people with both diagnoses.

A not entirely unrelated issue is that psychological treatments have rather more in common with surgical interventions than with pharmacological approaches, in that the very specific and individual nature of a person's psychological life is reflected both in the way in which an illness 'shows itself' and in the particular way in which a psychological treatment progresses. In a psychological treatment, therapists must work directly with an individual's psychological uniqueness, which in day-to-day clinical practice means that the rate, progress and specific focus of therapy will differ from individual to individual, even within the same diagnostic category. Similarly, the process of surgical intervention rests upon approaching the 'anatomical field' for each individual operation as a unique structure. The 'dose' of treatment, although important, is less relevant for psychological and surgical interventions than for drug treatments. This has two important implications for guidelines incorporating psychological treatments.

First, whereas pharmacological RCTs are designed to minimise the impact of individual differences, the design of psychological RCTs should focus less on the 'dose of therapy' and more on fitting the therapy to the specific psychological make-up and needs of the individual. To date, most psychological RCTs are modelled on the pharmacological RCT in which dose is given priority. For example, in the treatment of depression the number and length of treatment sessions given to each participant are much the same (e.g. CBT for depression: 16–20 weeks). RCTs of psychological interventions so designed, nevertheless, often show an average overall improvement for intervention groups, suggesting that we may be seriously underestimating the potential for this type of intervention.

Second, the skills and experience needed to undertake a psychological treatment effectively are also comparable to those needed for a surgical intervention, and the more complex illnesses and interventions require much higher levels of skill and experience. If this issue is to be effectively addressed, mental health guidelines will increasingly need to focus not just on conditions and interventions but also on the precise skills required to undertake interventions effectively.* Although RCTs of psychological

---

* Clinical practice guideline recommendations are designed to influence the behaviour of health professionals and evidence from health psychology suggests that recommendations must clearly delineate the precise behaviours required in order to bring about changes in behaviour. Such precise recommendations are often difficult to achieve in psychological treatments as the complexity of the interventions and the heterogeneity of the populations often make the generation of such precise recommendations difficult.

treatments increasingly use operationalised and 'manualised' therapeutic approaches, the skills of the therapists in a trial are rarely adequately described or indeed subject to any analysis.

Additional problems for guideline production relate to the course of mental health problems. Even very severe mental health problems, such as schizophrenia, do not always follow the same course or pattern as physical illnesses in that about one-quarter of people with schizophrenia get better for good, sometimes after many years of illness.[8] The methods of meta-analysis generally assume an illness has a more predictable course governed by the mechanisms that underlie the progression of an illness. The evaluation of treatments, at least in part, will depend upon the extent to which a treatment can alter that progression (for example, in the evaluation of aspirin or statins following a myocardial infarction). However, it is our impression that complex, heterogeneous and chronic physical conditions, such as multiple sclerosis, also show a variable and less predictable course, again presenting a challenge to standard meta-analytic techniques.

Although there is insufficient space to allow proper discussion, the placebo effect in trials of psychiatric drugs is often so large that specific pharmacological effects can be hard to identify, especially when given to people who fall into one of the larger, more heterogeneous diagnostic categories. Nowhere is this more apparent than in the treatment of depression.[9] From the depression guideline review, the evidence identified suggests that drug treatments, physical exercise and some types of supported self-help, when compared to waiting list controls, in the treatment of mild to moderate depression, all produce sizeable and comparable falls in depressive symptoms. However, when antidepressants are compared to placebo for the same diagnostic group, the effect size for antidepressants over and above that for placebo is not clinically significant.[9] In the context of recent concern over publication bias, particularly with regard to drug company-funded trials,[10,11] the possibility of some psychiatric drugs having no advantage, on average, over placebo may well prove challenging for future guidelines.

Finally, unlike other parts of medicine (except public health), psychiatrists not only have a responsibility to their patients, they also have the competing responsibility to protect the public and sometimes to use compulsion under the Mental Health Act to fulfil these responsibilities. The stigma experienced by those who use mental health services is arguably an important result of being subject to these different laws and practices. Whatever the cause of stigma, it has recently been suggested that the impact of stigma on the lives of people with some of the more severe mental illnesses now outweighs the impact of the illnesses themselves.[12] Having a good evidence base seems particularly important if a person is to be compulsorily treated. Correcting the stigma suffered by many people with mental health problems, and the impact this has on employment, relationships and indeed on the very fabric of people's lives, may require something more.

References

1 Dohrenwend BP (1990) The problem of validity in field studies of psycho-logical disorders revisited. *Psych Med.* **20**: 195–208.
2 Walsh T, Seidman S, Sysko R *et al.* (2002) Placebo response in studies of major depression: variable, substantial, and growing. *J Am Med Assoc.* **287**: 1840–7.
3 NICE (2002) *Schizophrenia: core interventions in the treatment and management of schizophrenia in primary and secondary care. NICE Clinical Guideline, No. 1.* NICE, London.
4 Eccles MP, Clapp Z, Grimshaw J *et al.* (1996) Developing valid guidelines: methodological and procedural issues from the North of England evidence based guideline development project. *Qual Health Care.* **5**: 44–50.
5 Kendall TJG, Pilling S, Barnes TRE *et al.* (2003) *Schizophrenia: full national clinical guideline on core interventions in primary and secondary care.* Gaskell, London.
6 World Health Organization (1992) *Tenth Revision of the International Classification of Diseases and Related Health Problems (ICD-10).* WHO, Geneva.
7 American Psychiatric Association (1994) *Diagnostic and Statistical Manual of Mental Disorders (DSM-IV)* (4e). American Psychiatric Press, Washington, DC.
8 Bleuler M (1978) The long-term course of schizophrenic psychosis. In: LC Wynne, RL Cromwell and S Matthysse (eds) *The Nature of Schizophrenia.* Wiley, New York.
9 Kirsch I, Moore T, Scoboria A *et al.* (2002) *The Emperor's New Drugs: an analysis of antidepressant medication data submitted to the US Food and Drug Administration. Prevention and Treatment.* **5**(23). www.journals.apa.org/prevention/volume5/pre0050023a.html
10 Lexchin J, Bero L, Djulbegovic B *et al.* (2003) Pharmaceutical industry sponsorship and research outcome and quality: systematic review. *BMJ.* **326**: 1167–70.
11 Melander H, Ahlqvist-Rastad J, Meijer G *et al.* (2003) Evidence b(i)ased medicine – selective reporting from studies sponsored by pharmaceutical industry: review of studies in new drug applications. *BMJ.* **326**: 1171–3.
12 Sartorius N (2002) Iatrogenic stigma of mental illness. *BMJ.* **324**: 1470–1.

Chapter 9

Using mental health guidelines in the NHS: views from a specialist mental health trust

Roger Paxton, Paula Whitty and Hugh Griffiths

The aim of this chapter is to explore how mental health organisations could use guidelines within their services. Our experience has mainly been in specialist mental health trusts, which is why we have focused on these within the chapter. However, mental health guidelines could be used in any organisation providing mental healthcare, from general primary care settings to multidisciplinary interface services, including services integrated with social care. We believe that the principles we highlight for specialist mental health trusts apply equally to other mental health services settings.

What sort of organisations are 'specialist mental health trusts'?

Following recent reorganisations within the NHS, most specialist mental health trusts are now fairly large in size and cover wide geographical areas, usually crossing several local government boundaries. Working with social services, wider local government, police, probation and other statutory and non-statutory agencies is an integral part of delivering mental health services. The range of services provided will usually include services for adults of working age and older people and will often include specialist mental health services for children and adolescents. Less widespread within specialist mental health trusts are forensic services and provision of services for people with learning disabilities. This all adds up to a complex environment for guidelines to operate in and one that is more complex than most physical healthcare environments. Mental healthcare is increasingly and intrinsically multiagency, with health and social care intertwined, and multisectoral, involving public and private, statutory and non-statutory sectors, housing, police and probation services. In addition to this, the involvement of service users and carers in service planning, delivery and evaluation is generally more advanced in mental health than physical healthcare. All of these groups are both stakeholders and partners in mental healthcare and the appropriate involvement of all must be considered if guidelines are to be implemented successfully.

Clinical practice guidelines and clinical governance in mental health trusts

Since 1999, all NHS organisations have been required to implement clinical governance. The basic components are a coherent approach to quality improvement, clear lines of accountability for clinical quality systems and effective processes for identifying and managing risk and addressing poor performance.[1] In the health service circular that accompanied the implementation of clinical governance, NHS trusts were required to ensure that 'evidence-based practice is supported and applied routinely in everyday practice' and that the 'clinical standards of National Service Frameworks and NICE recommendations are implemented'.[1] At about the same time, the Commission for Health Improvement (CHI) was established (now CHAI – the Commission for Healthcare Audit and Inspection), with the responsibility to 'independently scrutinise local clinical governance arrangements to support, promote and deliver high-quality services, through a rolling programme of local reviews of service providers'.[2] NHS trusts were to be subject to CHI clinical governance reviews approximately every three years, part of which includes assessment of the trust's 'clinical effectiveness' programme. CHI expected clinical effectiveness programmes to include a systematic approach to implementing clinical practice guidelines (CPGs). For example, CHI's guide to clinical governance reviews in mental health trusts specifically asks for evidence of the 'implementation and application of effective clinical practice, e.g. integrated care pathways; evidence-based guidelines for disease management'.[3]

What national policies are driving mental health trusts?

Aside from CHI clinical governance reviews, all NHS trusts are heavily performance managed, but not always on targets related to quality improvement or to the trust's own priorities. Mental health trusts are particularly focused on the Adult Mental Health National Service Framework (NSF), more recently on the Older People's NSF, and the Children's NSF will require increasing attention. Central directives to implement guidelines across services in mental health trusts have come from both the NSFs (for example, for depression and anxiety) and from NICE (*see* Chapter 6). Like other parts of the NHS, mental health trusts are also being actively encouraged to 'modernise', for example, to establish 'integrated care pathways' and undertake 'service redesign'.[4] Use of CPGs potentially helps to underpin these initiatives with evidence, as well as providing opportunities to implement CPGs within and across services and agencies.

What is the range of mental health guidance currently available?

As well as the mental health NICE guidelines (published or in preparation) described in Chapter 8, other sources of widely disseminated guidance in England include:

- NSF-related guidance, for example, the various Mental Health Policy Implementation Guides[5]
- the guidelines published by the Royal College of Psychiatrists (www.rcpsych.ac.uk)
- published integrated care pathways (for example, Dementia Care Pathways) (www.nelh.shef.ac.uk/nelh/kit/cps/paths.nsf/welcome?open).

However, not all of these guidelines are explicitly evidence based.

When there are large numbers of national and other external priorities, organisations can find it difficult to agree a manageable number of top priorities that command local support. One practical approach to this for guidelines is to focus on those areas where local priorities overlap with national 'givens' (for example, the NSF or NICE guidelines/guidance). A clear example for most mental health trusts currently would be schizophrenia.[6]

So how might you go about it? Practical ideas for mental health organisations

Since there is very little published about using guidelines in specialist mental health services, in this section of the chapter we present two case studies from our experience. One is currently in progress and highly topical as it examines the issues expected to be involved in implementing the NICE schizophrenia guideline[6] through an integrated care pathway. The other looks at what can be learned for guidelines implementation from the first mental health 'collaborative' project in the UK, which aimed to improve acute inpatient care.

Case study 1: What issues does a trust need to take into account when planning an integrated care pathway based on the NICE Schizophrenia Guideline?

There is considerable enthusiasm in British mental health services for the potential benefits of emerging CPGs. The NICE Schizophrenia Guideline is widely seen as exemplary for its thoroughness, accessibility and reason-ableness. However, there is equally widespread uncertainty and some concern regarding the practicalities of implementing CPGs in general and the NICE Schizophrenia Guideline in particular. Some of the issues surrounding this are as follows.

1 Workload and time issues (and in particular how to engage the staff who need to be actively involved).
2 The skills needed to implement guidelines (what kinds of project management skills, educational and other guidelines implementation skills are needed and where can they be found?).
3 Organising the overall implementation into a series of manageable tasks (what should the tasks be and how should they be sequenced and managed?).
4 Engaging the organisation and wider health community (who needs to be informed and involved and how?).
5 Resource implications (what resources are needed for implementation and what, if anything, can be done using only existing resources?). This includes organisation-wide resources such as electronic health information systems.

These issues probably apply across all fields of healthcare, but mental health presents additional implementation challenges, with most services extensively multiagency and with high and quite proper expectations of close user and carer involvement adding further to the complexity of the environment.

At the time of writing, we are only part way through our project to implement an integrated care pathway based on the NICE Schizophrenia Guideline, so much of what we describe relates to the project planning stage. From our interpretation of the organisational change literature,[7] we identified five broad stages to implement guidelines in our setting, which we used as a framework for the project (Box 9.1).

Box 9.1: Project framework

1 Describing current services and pathways
2 Comparing them with those in the guideline
3 Identifying gaps and variances
4 Specifying realistic services and pathways that are as compliant as possible with the guideline within the local context
5 Planning staged implementation

It was immediately apparent that the task of developing an integrated care pathway for schizophrenia in our trust was very large, because of the number of services that need to be involved in the care of this client group. To make worthwhile progress in a reasonable timescale, additional project management support was needed and the work outlined here (estimated to take a year) is being led by an experienced external project manager with a full-time assistant psychologist supporting her and two senior members of staff steering and overseeing the work. The activities in more detail at each stage are described below.

1 Describe current services and pathways

To describe current service elements and pathways required the various stakeholder groups to be identified. These groups also needed to be involved so that the description is not isolated from the subsequent change tasks as new pathways are to be planned and implemented. As we have not yet completed the work, we cannot comment on how easy or difficult this task is; for example, whether pathways are always obvious and whether people agree on what they are. However, even at this stage, the process has already revealed considerable variation in practice across the trust (for example, the availability of family therapy), which will clearly need to be addressed as part of the project.

Stakeholders are service users and carers and all of the services, professions and agencies who do or should contribute to the care of people with schizophrenia. For us, this amounts to a substantial group of people. In order to allow them to work together productively we established a Project Board, comprising service user and carer representatives, the project manager and the most senior management and clinical representatives from the trust. The Board has overall authority and responsibility for the project. The main functions of the Board are to establish and make use of the commitment of all the stakeholder organisations. Reporting to the Board is the Project Management Group, comprising the two senior clinical staff responsible for the project and the part-time seconded project manager. The Board and Project Management Group consult with a much wider stakeholder group, using open forum meetings, regular project newsletters and Internet updates and questions. From this consultation we aim to sustain the commitment and motivation of individuals at various levels within the stakeholder organisations. From the wider stakeholder group, topic working groups are currently being established to work on fairly short-term tasks, reporting back to both the stakeholder group and Board.

We agreed that the description of current service elements should include information on numbers of people receiving the key treatment interventions included in the NICE guidelines. Cognitive behaviour therapy (CBT), family interventions and prescribing patterns are central here. Experience from elsewhere suggests that a useful framework for this description is 'process mapping'.[8] According to this framework, the description of services and pathways needs to be supplemented by a similar description of communication arrangements. So we are in the process of identifying how referral guidance and other information *should* flow between services and how it *actually* flows.

We also plan to collect descriptive information on outcomes. We expect this to consist mainly of service intermediate outcomes, for example, activity data on patient flows between services, duration of inpatient stays, bed occupancy levels and so on. Where outcome information is available (for example, routinely collected clinical rating scales), we will try to collect it.

2 Compare actual pathways with the NICE guidelines

As well as trying not to isolate the descriptive stage from the change process, we aim not to separate it from evaluation. We are planning to make the baseline data outlined here the first stage of a formative evaluation process. We see stakeholder involvement here, as elsewhere, as essential. As engagement is a step towards motivation for change, we will be noting the perceptions of different stakeholder groups on the gaps and variances. At this stage we expect issues of guideline coverage to arise. For example, in the case of the Schizophrenia Guideline, there has already been vigorous discussion on how to deal with services for other forms of psychosis that clearly overlap with those for schizophrenia. There has also been discussion on how to deal with interventions currently provided but not covered by the guideline, for example, some of the social interventions delivered by occupational therapists. We have decided with our stakeholders to address these issues of coverage by sticking as closely as possible to the coverage of the guideline for the duration of the project. Then, after the project is completed, we shall consider the extent to which our redesigned pathways are also applicable or easily modifiable to encompass other psychoses and other interventions.

3 Identify gaps and variances

This stage, which will begin shortly, will describe and evaluate the importance of the differences identified. We anticipate that this will be very important in relation to establishing motivation for change. We want to identify how particular stakeholder groups would benefit from closing a particular gap and what disadvantages might arise, amounting to obstacles to change. Positive and negative motivational factors will be identified for different groups through their involvement at this stage, recorded for use in subsequent steps.

4 Specify realistic NICE-compliant services and pathways

It is likely that we will need to compromise, so involving all stakeholders in realistic improvements will, we hope, be another step towards effective motivation for change. Realistic services must take account of financial constraints, concentrating on service functions rather than particular structures, as described in the Policy Implementation Guides.[5] Also they must take account of the local context. In our case, one of the three major localities in our large trust is mainly rural and there is increasing acknowledgement of the need for rural variants of models for the new functional mental health services.

We expect that analysing process maps produced earlier will reveal opportunities for improvement in some elements of care pathways that will remain and this has been extremely useful within the Acute Inpatient Mental Health Collaborative, as Case Study 2 illustrates. The end point at this stage will comprise detailed descriptions of the functions and components of the service elements, following as closely as possible those described in the guideline and a similar description of the service processes and pathways between elements.

5 Plan staged implementation

We expect that the local context will provide the most important set of factors that determine the stages and timescales for implementing new pathways. Funding pressures and opportunities are likely to be one of the main issues for us. For instance, there is growing evidence that effective crisis resolution services reduce inpatient bed usage and can lead to significant bed reductions, thus allowing transfers of funding.[9] Similarly, from the evidence, effective assertive outreach teams should relieve the pressure on community mental health teams,[10] which might allow funding transfers or redirection to deliver services differently in accordance with the new pathways. External pressures are likely to impact on the local context through the timescales for NSF targets and the availability of central funding. A current example is the requirement to deliver early interventions in psychosis, which will require us to develop these services at an early stage of implementation. Taking account of these factors, the end point of this stage will be a set of goals for implementation; that is, a plan with timescales, notes on responsibilities for different staff at different stages and notes on any external factors required to proceed with implementation at any stage.

6 Accountability, monitoring and evaluation

At the outset, we clarified the accountability and reporting arrangements for the project, with a lead clinician and lead director reporting on progress to the trust's Clinical Governance Committee every three months. Our aim is to evaluate the project according to whether its original goals have been achieved. In order to do this, these goals will need to be translated into measurable outcomes, to enable us to answer the following questions.

- Has the service been set up as intended?
- Is it functioning as intended?
- Is it achieving its intended outcomes?

7 Summary

In summary, from our local analysis and from our experience so far, implementation of an integrated care pathway based on the NICE Schizophrenia Guideline will be a complex process, mirroring the complexity of specialist mental healthcare. We are adopting a project management approach to this and, in our view, regard dedicated project management time and expertise as essential components. Full involvement and engagement of all the stakeholders will be vital at every stage of the project, including its monitoring and evaluation.

Case study 2: Service redesign – the experience of the Acute Inpatient Mental Health Collaborative and the potential role of clinical practice guidelines

A wide range of guides are now available on how to carry out service redesign and re-engineering.[4] One of the processes underlying these approaches is a continuous quality improvement tool known as the 'Plan Do Study Act' (PDSA) cycle.[4,8] One of us (HG) has experience as the 'clinical lead' in a mental health 'collaborative' project across 37 multidisciplinary teams, which incorporated PDSA methodology.

The former Trent and Northern and Yorkshire NHS Executive offices, together with the Northern Centre for Mental Health, jointly commissioned a 15-month Mental Health Collaborative which commenced in October 2000. The aim of the project was to improve service users' experiences of acute inpatient care and achieve better outcomes throughout the process of admission, stay and discharge. Almost all mental health trusts in the two former regions participated. Based on the Institute of Healthcare Improvement methodology,[8] a Collaborative is a process for bringing about change by supporting clinical teams to try out small changes in order to improve services. Working on a set of change ideas produced by an invited 'reference group', all clinical project teams met at a series of learning sessions in order to compare experiences and measure whether their changes had resulted in positive outcomes. One of the most important features of this Collaborative was the active engagement of service users within the whole process.

Although the Mental Health Collaborative project did not set out to implement CPGs, some of the lessons learnt from the project are very relevant to guidelines implementation. There are several opportunities in the PDSA process to apply CPGs (including several points at which a thorough search for evidence needs to be carried out):

- following mapping of the service user's journey – matching what actually happens in the service to the best available evidence (including relevant CPGs) as one of the ways of identifying areas for change
- reviewing existing audit data against CPGs to help identify needs for change
- using CPGs to derive measurement criteria/standards in the areas of change agreed
- the CPGs themselves may be a tool to support change, for example, where one of the priorities identified for change is an area of clinical practice for which a CPG is available.

One of the key points is that, used in the Collaborative context, the change to be put in place is service user (rather than guideline) driven, but still promotes the best use of evidence.

Conversely, the Collaborative methodology is a technique for implementing specific aspects of change required by guidelines, particularly where these are practical, local organisational changes. However, even quite wide and complex changes were achieved by the Collaborative as the project progressed and teams gained confidence, for example, introducing care pathways and changing staff roles.

Having established project starting positions on the improvement measures agreed by the 'reference group', project teams prioritised areas for action and agreed their initial PDSA cycles. Between January and December 2001, the project teams collectively generated 2070 PDSA cycles and implemented 377 permanent changes. The range and size of changes varied widely between teams (for examples, *see* Box 9.2).

Box 9.2: Examples of changes in service following PDSA cycles

- Published service user information booklets/leaflets
- Streamlined risk assessment and single multidisciplinary team assessment tools
- Integrated care pathways introduced
- Improved therapeutic inputs
- Better discharge communication systems in place

Some of the reflections on what made this process work included:[11]

- placing the service user at the centre of the process
- the most valuable tool in the collection of data was mapping the service user's journey
- the concept of building small changes into large improvement
- the methodology was seen as useful because it encouraged participation and ownership. Project teams reported that they felt empowered and motivated to initiate change.

One conclusion drawn by the project leaders was that the Mental Health Collaborative has made a 'significant move away from the "hero-innovator" towards a more empowering means of creating sustainable change through the utilisation of shared perspectives and of jointly owned goals'.[11]

In our view, the lessons from the Collaborative project are highly relevant to guidelines implementation within our trust and we are attempting to apply them to the NICE Schizophrenia Guideline (as in the first case study). For example, allowing staff and service users to drive the projects together; beginning by mapping the user's current journey before attempting any change in services; applying the guideline to this map, to identify the service changes required; and trying to identify 'bite-size' changes that can be implemented as a programme of change over a realistic period of time.

Conclusions

Drawing on our experience from both case studies (Box 9.3), guidelines implementation in a specialist mental health trust is a complex process, mirroring the complexity of specialist mental healthcare, which takes place in a multiagency and multisectoral environment. We believe that a project management approach should be adopted and that dedicated project management time and expertise are essential components. Full involvement and engagement of all the stakeholders are vital at every stage, including monitoring and evaluation. From the Collaborative project's experience in particular, implementation of a guideline should be broken up into a stepwise programme of small, achievable service changes and both staff and service users should be empowered to be able to get on with making these changes happen.

Box 9.3: Key points from the case studies

- Specialist mental healthcare takes place in a complex multiagency and multisectoral environment.
- Service user and carer involvement in the planning, delivery and evaluation of care is generally more advanced than in physical healthcare. Their involvement in guidelines implementation is pivotal.
- The guidelines agenda has mainly been driven by the NSFs (notably for working-age adults) but is now also being driven from NICE.
- From our experience, guidelines implementation in this complex environment requires wide stakeholder involvement, a project management approach and a stepwise programme of small, achievable service changes.

References

1 NHS Executive (1999) *Clinical Governance: quality in the new NHS. Health Service Circular 1999/065*. The Stationery Office, London.

2 NHS Executive (1998) *A First Class Service*. The Stationery Office, London.

3 Commission for Health Improvement (2003) *Guide to the Clinical Governance Review Process in Mental Health Services*. CHI, London.
www.chi.nhs.uk/eng/cgr/mental_health/cgr_guide_mh.doc

4 NHS Modernisation Agency. *Improvement Leaders Guides*.
www.modern.nhs.uk/improvementguides/

5 Department of Health (2001) *Policy Implementation Guides*. HMSO, London.

6 NICE (2002) *Schizophrenia: core interventions in the treatment and management of schizophrenia in primary and secondary care. NICE Clinical Guideline, No. 1*. NICE, London.

7 Iles V and Sutherland K (2002) *Managing Change in the NHS. Organisational change: a review for healthcare managers, professionals and researchers*. National Co-ordinating Centre for NHS Service Delivery and Organisation R&D, London.

8 Berwick DM (1989) Continuous improvement as an ideal in healthcare. *N Engl J Med.* **320**: 53–6.

9 Kennedy P (2003) *More Than the Sum of All the Parts: improving the whole system with crisis resolution and home treatment*. Northern Centre for Mental Health, York.

10 Priebe S, Bebbington P, Burns T *et al.* (2003) Assertive outreach teams in London: patient characteristics and outcomes. Pan-London assertive outreach study, Part 3. *Br J Psych.* **183**: 148–54.

11 Robert G, Hardacre J, Locock L *et al.* (2003) Redesigning mental health services: lessons on user involvement from the Mental Health Collaborative. *Health Expectations.* **6**(1): 60–71.

Chapter 10

Using mental health guidelines in primary care: the example of depression management

Paul Walters, Simon Gilbody and Andre Tylee

Over 90% of patients with mental health problems are treated in primary care alone.[1,2] Depression is by far the most common mental health problem treated in primary care. Studies examining consecutive attendees in general practice have estimated that between 5 and 15% suffer from major depression.[3,4] In a practice list of 2000 patients it has been calculated that 60 to 100 people will suffer from depression, 70 to 80 with anxiety and 50 to 60 with a situational disturbance.[5]

Depression in the primary care setting poses a considerable burden not only on the individual and their family but also on primary care services and economically on the wider society. By the year 2020 it has been estimated that depression will be the leading cause of disability after ischaemic heart disease.[6] Patients suffering from depression consult two to three times more often than the general population, which may explain why up to 30% of consultations held in primary care concern such problems.[7]

Despite the clinical and economic burden associated with depression, there is substantial evidence that depression within primary care settings is poorly recognised or sub-optimally managed.[2,8,9] There is therefore an opportunity to improve individual patient outcomes and to reduce the burden of suffering at a population level through improvements in the quality of care. Guidelines are an important and increasingly advocated mechanism to improve healthcare quality. The purpose of this chapter is to provide an overview of the research evidence to support the effective implementation of guidelines for depression in primary care and to discuss the implications of this research for practitioners and decision makers in primary care settings.

Depression guidelines in primary care

The National Service Framework (NSF) for Mental Health in England has set out the national standards that services delivering mental healthcare must meet.[10] Within this framework, depression has been identified as a priority area for guideline development. Currently the National Institute for Clinical Excellence (NICE) is preparing clinical practice guidelines for the management of depression, which will have particular relevance to primary care. Complementing the work of NICE, the National Institute for Mental Health in England (NIMHE), as part of the Modernisation Agency of the Department of Health, has developed a Primary Care Programme.[11,12] This programme could have an important role in aiding the dissemination and implementation of guidelines in primary care, working within its aims of improving the fundamentals of primary mental healthcare and facilitating innovative practice.

The programme has five proposed areas consistent with current policy to address the agendas of the NHS Plan and NSF for Mental Health. These are: staff development, commissioning and developing effective partnerships, developing the primary care user perspective, integrating care for people with severe mental health problems and research and development. Eight regional development centres have been established to ensure the five areas are being developed nationally and a national programme manager has been appointed to co-ordinate and implement the programme plan.

The use of depression guidelines in primary care

Early UK primary care depression guidelines were developed as a joint campaign organised by the Royal College of Psychiatrists with the Royal College of General Practitioners in 1992.[13] Other early and influential attempts at developing evidence-based guidelines were those from the US Agency for Health Care and Policy Research (AHCPR).[14] However, a general concern has emerged about the potential for guidelines, by themselves, to improve depression management in primary care.[15]

Much has been learned in recent years about the effectiveness and efficiency of guideline dissemination and implementation strategies. Systematic review methods have been applied to the guidelines literature, initially through the work of Grimshaw and Russell[16] and more recently through the use of methods developed within the Cochrane Effective Practice and Organisation of Care (EPOC) group.[17] Evidence, in the form of potentially rigorous evaluations of guideline dissemination and implementation programmes (RCTs, controlled clinical trials, controlled before and after studies, and interrupted time series analyses), has been sought and subjected to critical evaluation. These methods were recently adopted to review the effectiveness of guideline implementation strategies for depression in primary care settings by Gilbody and colleagues[18–20] and form the most up-to-date and rigorous summary of the existing research. The results of this review are informative in that they tell us which implementation strategies work for depression in primary care settings and which do not.

Effective strategies

Guidelines, and strategies to implement them, have been used as a method of *decision support* for clinicians in a number of successful interventions. Guideline implementation strategies were varied and often complex and included active dissemination and clinician education – such as academic detailing, peer review and the use of opinion leaders. Guideline implementation strategies targeted at the overall recognition and management of depression were only successful when educational interventions were accompanied by complex organisational interventions – such as nurse case management,[21] collaborative care,[22] a Depression Management Programme[23] or intensive quality improvement.[24] Case examples of these successful strategies are described in turn below.

Collaborative care

Two major US studies by Katon and colleagues[25,26] used a population-based approach to improve the *delivery of care* for those with already recognised depression.[27] Intensified care incorporating patient education, shared care between the primary care physician, psychiatrist and psychologist were associated with improved treatment adherence and patient recovery rates. This approach resulted in a lower overall cost per patient successfully treated. A sustained improvement in the management of depressive disorders was not seen beyond the period of enhanced organisational care,[28] suggesting that clinician education alone was not sufficient in maintaining change.

A supplementary intervention, targeted at those at high risk of recurrence of depression following acute-phase treatment, showed improved medication concordance (odds ratio [OR] 2.08, 95% confidence interval [CI] 1.41–3.06) and depression at 12 months.[29] A more recent study[30] has also shown that collaborative care can be extended to late life depression, where patient education, case management and problem-solving therapy were associated with improved medication concordance (OR 3.45, 95%CI 2.71–4.38) and depression at 12 months (OR 2.03, 95%CI 1.60–2.57).

Stepped collaborative care

A related intervention,[22,31] which aimed to improve the *delivery of care*, offered enhanced care for patients not responding to usual care by a primary care physician. A combination of patient education, clinician education meetings, automated pharmacy data and enhanced collaborative management by a psychiatrist in a primary care setting (advice and direct patient review) resulted in enhanced medication concordance (relative risk [RR] 1.43, 95%CI 1.16–1.78, numbers needed to treat [NNT] = 5) and recovery (RR 1.42, 95%CI 1.02–2.03, NNT = 8) at six months and persisted at 28-month follow-up.

Quality improvement

Two large randomised studies[24,32–35] examined a complex package of care, *quality improvement*, targeted at recognition (through screening) and management of depression. This complex organisational and educational intervention involved patient screening by questionnaire, clinician education, opinion leaders, patient-specific reminders, nurse case management (*see* below) and integration with specialist care. Quality improvement was targeted at either improved concordance with medication (*QI meds*) or improved uptake of cognitive behavioural therapy (*QI therapy*). Both interventions were effective in improving both medication concordance (p < 0.001) and depression (p = 0.03) over six and 12 months, although the benefit for depression outcomes had disappeared at 24-month follow-up.

Case management

An almost uniform feature of positive studies was the incorporation of some form of *case management*, usually by primary care nurses, to improve the *delivery of care*.[21,23,29,33,36–38] In some studies, nurse involvement was of low intensity and involved little more than brief medication counselling[38] or support over the phone.[36] In others, nurse case management was a core ingredient of an effective complex strategy.[21,23,31,33] For example, in the QuEST study,[21,39] non-psychiatrically trained practice nurses were given training in the management of depression and they provided a level of ongoing support and monitored therapy, outpatient attendance and treatment response according to well-established algorithms. Nurse case management was delivered solely over the phone using 10-minute phone calls ('*Nurse Telehealthcare*') in one study,[36] which showed improved outcomes for depression. In an important UK study[38] it was demonstrated that two brief 20-minute follow-up sessions to discuss medication could substantially enhance concordance (OR 2.7, 95%CI 1.6–4.8, NNT 4) and depression outcome was improved in a subset of patients with major depression.[38]

Pharmacist-delivered prescribing information and patient education

Clinician education on prescribing (but not recognition and other management), delivered by pharmacists to groups of physicians, resulted in improved prescribing of antidepressants amongst patients over 60 (RR 0.55, 95%CI 0.33–0.92).[40] A large UK trial of primary care physician educational outreach (academic detailing)[41] delivered by pharmacists,[42] which included advice on antidepressant prescribing, showed a non-significant increase of 4% in the percentage of patients treated according to medication guidelines.

Strategies not shown to be effective in depression

Educational strategies

An important negative and well-designed UK study (The Hampshire Depression Project) involved a well-developed clinician education and guideline implementation strategy that was well received in primary care.[43,44] Education involved videos, written materials, small group teaching sessions and role-play and was delivered by a multidisciplinary team. However, there was no organisational support to enhance individual patient care. The intervention had no impact on either recognition rates for depression (sensitivity OR 1.00, 95%CI 0.73–1.37; specificity OR 0.97, 95%CI 0.70–1.34) or clinical improvement (OR 1.23, 95%CI 0.84–1.79).[45] Less complex guideline implementation strategies were also negative[46,47] or showed mixed results.[48]

An influential positive GP educational study using local opinion leaders, conducted on the Swedish island of Gotland in the 1980s, using an interrupted time series analysis, showed an apparent reduction in suicide rates and an increase in antidepressant prescription.[49,50] However, this was a weak methodological design, subject to many biases and errors of analysis, including a unit of analysis error. While there are examples of trials showing education influencing prescribing,[40,42] the other outcomes of the Gotland study have never been replicated using more methodologically robust designs. Other educational strategies were largely negative; for example, studies of clinician education, even when accompanied by audit and feedback or academic detailing,[51] showed no impact on depression, quality of life or concordance with medication. Educational meetings, whilst improving clinicians' knowledge and attitudes about depression,[52] had no impact on practice or depression outcomes.[53]

Effective use of depression guidelines by primary care trusts and practices

Evidence suggests that to maximise the probability of clinical practice guidelines being implemented, they need to be adapted with due consideration of local circumstances.[16] At a local level primary care trusts (PCTs) play a vital role. PCTs need to provide guidelines that reflect local needs and promote local ownership, but which are based on nationally produced guidelines (such as the forthcoming NICE depression guidelines). Currently PCTs have a crucial role in overseeing audit, monitoring performance indicators and clinical governance. This needs to be developed further so that they not only monitor and identify local variations in care provision but also address the greater challenge of promoting professional change once such variability has been identified. Targeting the implementation of clinical practice guidelines on practices that are under-performing may be one way to rectify such variations in care.

Despite the disappointing results of guideline dissemination and educational initiatives alone in improving the management of depression in primary care, there is now a substantial evidence base to suggest that clinical practice guidelines can be effective in primary care when used within the context of enhanced care processes and organisational restructuring. This has led von Korff and Goldberg to suggest that efforts to improve the primary care management of depression should focus on low-cost case management and close liaison between the GP, case manager and mental health specialist.[15] Local guidelines could also be adapted from the national guidelines for the roles of the 1000 new primary care graduate workers, who are now being employed in England,[54] and other mental health primary care workers such as the gateway or liaison workers.[55] These workers are ideally placed to act as 'case managers' in the effective management of depression[15] and to work within 'collaborative care' models. The value of collaborative care models is recognised within the draft NICE guidelines, where 'enhanced care for depression' is strongly supported.

Practices and PCTs might also consider how they might implement organisational changes in the delivery of care, such as 'stepped care' approaches. The successful implementation of stepped care will depend on the development and reconfiguration of the relationship between primary and secondary care services. In some localities, existing relationships at the primary/secondary care interface will be good and stepped care might represent a refinement of an already good and collaborative relationship. However, in others, where there is fragmentation between services, approaches such as stepped care will require substantial reconfiguration of roles and boundaries that are potentially more difficult to achieve. The commissioning role within PCTs presents a substantial lever in facilitating the organisational changes required to implement successful guidelines. A further financial incentive has been established within the newly agreed General Medical Services (GMS) contract, where depression is one of 12 clinical areas singled out for extra payments under the National Enhanced Services scheme. Practices will receive payments of £100 per patient in receipt of care that is in some way 'enhanced' and this should ideally be based upon effective models of case management and collaborative care.

Clinical practice guidelines need the associated resources for good dissemination and implementation. PCTs therefore have to provide the resources necessary for the development of methods that allow for organisational development. Without a change in the whole process of care it is unlikely that clinical practice guidelines will effect improved clinical outcomes. The priority for primary care trusts therefore should not be the creation of more and more guidelines but rather adapting nationally accepted guidelines for local use by hard-pressed primary care professionals and using the robust evidence presented above to achieve successful implementation.

Conclusions

Clinical practice guidelines are now part of the landscape in clinical medicine and are likely to become an increasingly dominant part of the vista. Primary care has been a particular focus for these guidelines. However, the majority of evidence to date suggests that, in primary care, depression guidelines and educational initiatives alone do little to improve the provision of care. The use of clinical practice guidelines, especially in primary care, has been controversial and their relevance to primary care has been questioned. There is also a fear that they may be used politically. What is clear is that guidelines can be implemented successfully when they are part of a care package and that this can be done cost-effectively. Primary care manages the vast majority of mental health problems, of which depression is the most common. The challenge for the future is developing the organisational structures, professional and personal cultures within which best practice evidence-based care can be provided, using guidelines to achieve a service in which patients and their carers can expect the same standard of high-quality care irrespective of where they seek help. This is unlikely to be achieved by a top-down approach alone. Primary care trusts, guided by organisations such as NIMHE, using clinical practice guidelines developed nationally by organisations such as NICE but adapted by stakeholders to meet local needs, may be the most successful way of improving the management of depression in primary care.

References

1   Shepherd M, Cooper B, Brown AC *et al.* (1996) *Psychiatric Illness in General Practice.* Oxford University Press, Oxford.
2   Goldberg D and Huxley P (1980) *Mental Illness in the Community.* Tavistock, London.
3   Freeling P, Rao BM, Paykel ES *et al.* (1985) Unrecognised depression in general practice. *BMJ.* **290**: 1880–3.
4   Tiemens BG, Ormel J and Simon GE (1996) Occurrence, recognition, and outcome of psychological disorders in primary care. *Am J Psych.* **153**: 636–44.
5   Strathdee G and Jenkins R (1996) Purchasing mental health for primary care. In: G Thornicroft and G Strathdee (eds) *Commissioning Mental Health Services.* HMSO, London.
6   Murray CJ and Lopez AD (1996) *The Global Burden of Disease: a comprehensive assessment of mortality and disability from disease, injuries and risk factors in 1990.* Harvard School of Public Health on behalf of the World Bank, Boston, MA.
7   Lepine JP, Gaskpar M, Mendlewicz J *et al.* (1997) Depression in the community: the first pan-European study, DEPRES (Depression Research in European Society). *Int Clin Psychopharm.* **12**: 19–29.

8 Kessler D, Lloyd K, Lewis G *et al.* (1999) Cross sectional study of symptom attribution and recognition of depression and anxiety in primary care. *BMJ.* **318**: 436–40.

9 Simon G and von Korff M (1995) Recognition and management of depression in primary care. *Arch Fam Med.* **4**: 99–105.

10 Secretary of State for Health (1999) *National Service Framework – Mental Health*. HMSO, London.

11 Tylee A (2003) The Primary Care Programme of the National Institute for Mental Health in England (NIMHE). *Primary Care Mental Health* **1**: 1–3.

12 Department of Health (2002) *First Year Strategy for NIMHE*. NIMHE/Department of Health, Leeds.

13 Paykel ES and Priest RG (1992) Recognition and management of depression in general practice: consensus statement. *BMJ.* **305**: 1198–202.

14 Agency for Health Care Policy Research (1993) *Depression in Primary Care*. US Department of Health and Human Services, Washington, DC.

15 von Korff M and Goldberg D (2001) Improving outcomes of depression: the whole process of care needs to be enhanced. *BMJ.* **323**: 948–9.

16 Grimshaw JM and Russell IT (1993) Effect of clinical guidelines on medical practice. A systematic review of rigorous evaluations. *Lancet.* **342**: 1317–22.

17 Bero L *et al.* (1998) The Cochrane Effective Practice and Organisation of Care Group (EPOC) Module. In: *The Cochrane Library, Issue 4*. Update Software, Oxford.

18 Gilbody SM, Whitty P, Grimshaw J *et al.* (2003) Improving the detection and management of depression in primary care. *Qual Saft Health Care.* **12**: 149–55.

19 Gilbody S, Whitty P, Grimshaw J *et al.* (2002) Improving the recognition and management of depression in primary care. *Effect Health Care Bull.* **7**. University of York, York.

20 Gilbody S, Whitty P, Grimshaw J *et al.* (2003) Educational and organizational interventions to improve the management of depression in primary care: a systematic review. *J Am Med Assoc.* **289**: 3145–51.

21 Rost K, Nutting PA, Smith J *et al.* (2001) Improving depression outcomes in community primary care practice: a randomised trial of the QuEST intervention. *J Gen Int Med.* **16**: 143–9.

22 Lin EH, von Korff M, Russo J *et al.* (2000) Can depression treatment in primary care reduce disability? A stepped care approach. *Arch Fam Med.* **9**: 1052–8.

23 Katzelnick DJ, Simon GF, Pearson SD *et al.* (2000) Randomized trial of a depression management program in high utilizers of medical care. *Arch Fam Med.* **9**: 345–51.

24 Sherbourne CD, Wells KB, Duan N *et al.* (2001) Long-term effectiveness of disseminating quality improvement for depression in primary care. *Arch Gen Psych.* **58**: 696–703.

25 Katon W, Robinson P, von Korff M *et al.* (1996) A multifaceted intervention to improve treatment of depression in primary care. *Arch Gen Psych.* **53**: 924–32.

26 Katon W, von Korff M, Lin E *et al.* (1995) Collaborative management to achieve treatment guidelines. Impact on depression in primary care. *J Am Med Assoc.* **273**: 1026–31.

27 Katon W, von Korff M, Lin E *et al.* (1997) Population-based care of depression: effective disease management strategies to decrease prevalence. *Gen Hosp Psych.* **19**: 169–78.

28 Lin EH, Katon WJ, Simon GF *et al.* (1997) Achieving guidelines for the treatment of depression in primary care: is physician education enough? *Med Care.* **35**: 831–42.

29 Katon W, Rutter C, Ludman EJ *et al.* (2001) A randomised trial of relapse prevention of depression in primary care. *Arch Gen Psych.* **58**: 241–7.

30 Unutzer J, Katon W, Callahan CM *et al.* (2002) Collaborative care management of late-life depression in the primary care setting: a randomised controlled trial. *J Am Med Assoc.* **288**: 2836–45.

31 Katon W, von Korff M, Lin E *et al.* (1999) Stepped collaborative care for primary care patients with persistent symptoms of depression: a randomised trial. *Arch Gen Psych.* **56**: 1109–15.

32 Rubenstein LV, Jackson-Triche M, Unutzer J *et al.* (1999) Evidence-based care for depression in managed primary care practices. *Health Aff (Millwood).* **18**: 89–105.

33 Wells KA, Sherbourne C, Schoenbaum M *et al.* (2000) Impact of disseminating quality improvement programmes for depression in managed primary care: a randomised controlled trial. *J Am Med Assoc.* **283**: 212–20.

34 Unutzer J, Rubenstein L, Katon WJ *et al.* (2001) Two-year effects of quality improvement programs on medication management for depression. *Arch Gen Psych.* **58**: 935–42.

35 Schoenbaum M, Unutzer J, Sherbourne C *et al.* (2001) Cost-effectiveness of practice-initiated quality improvement for depression: results of a randomised controlled trial. *J Am Med Assoc.* **286**: 1325–30.

36 Hunkeler EM, Meresman JF, Hargreaves WA *et al.* (2000) Efficacy of nurse telehealthcare and peer support in augmenting treatment of depression in primary care. *Arch Fam Med.* **9**: 700–8.

37 Simon GE, von Korff M, Rutter C *et al.* (2000) Randomised trial of monitoring, feedback, and management of care by telephone to improve treatment of depression in primary care. *BMJ.* **320**: 550–4.

38 Peveler R, George C, Kinmonth AL *et al.* (1999) Effect of antidepressant drug counselling and information leaflets on adherence to drug treatment in primary care: randomised controlled trial. *BMJ.* **319**: 612–5.

39 Rost K, Nutting PA, Smith J *et al.* (2000) Designing and implementing a primary care intervention trial to improve the quality and outcome of care for major depression. *Gen Hosp Psych.* **22**: 66–77.

40 van Eijk ME, Avorn J, Porsius AJ *et al.* (2001) Reducing prescribing of highly anticholinergic antidepressants for elderly people: randomised trial of group versus individual academic detailing. *BMJ.* **322**: 654–7.

41 Soumerai SB and Avorn J (1990) Principles of educational outreach ('academic detailing') to improve clinical decision making. *J Am Med Assoc.* **26**: 549–56.

42 Freemantle N, Nazareth I, Eccles M *et al.* (2002) A randomised controlled trial of the effect of educational outreach by community pharmacists on prescribing in UK general practice. *Br J Gen Pract.* **52**: 290–5.

43 Thompson C, Kinmonth J, Stevens L *et al.* (2000) Effects of a clinical practice guideline and practice-based education on detection and outcome of depression in primary care: Hampshire Depression Project randomised controlled trial. *Lancet.* **355**: 50–7.

44 Kendrick T, Stevens L, Bryant A *et al.* (2001) Hampshire depression project: changes in the process of care and cost consequences. *Br J Gen Pract.* **51**: 911–13.

45 Peveler R and Kendrick T (2001) Treatment delivery and guidelines in primary care. *Br Med Bull.* **57**: 193–206.

46 Wilkinson G, Allen P and Marshall E (1993) The role of the practice nurse in the management of depression in general practice: treatment adherence to antidepressant medication. *Psychol Med.* **23**: 229–37.

47 Mann A, Blizard R and Murray J (1998) An evaluation of practice nurses working with general practitioners to treat people with depression. *Br J Gen Pract.* **48**: 875–9.

48 Baker R, Reddish S, Robertson N *et al.* (2001) Randomised controlled trial of tailored strategies to implement guidelines for the management of patients with depression in general practice. *Br J Gen Pract.* **51**: 737–41.

49 Rutz W, von Knorring L and Walinder J (1989) Frequency of suicide on Gotland after systematic postgraduate education for general practitioners. *Acta Psychiatr Scand.* **80**: 151–4.

50 Rutz W, von Knorring L and Walinder J (1992) Long-term effects of an educational program for general practitioners given by the Swedish Committee for the Prevention and Treatment of Depression. *Acta Psychiatr Scand.* **85**: 83–8.

51 Brown JB, Shye D, McFarland BH *et al.* (2000) Controlled trials of CQI and academic detailing to implement a clinical practice guideline for depression. *J Qual Improv.* **26**: 39–54.

52 Andersen SM and Harthorn BH (1990) Changing the psychiatric knowledge of primary care physicians: the effects of a brief intervention on clinical diagnosis and treatment. *Gen Hosp Psych.* **12**: 177–90.

53 Worrall G, Angel J, Chaulk P *et al.* (1999) Effectiveness of an educational strategy to improve family physicians' detection and management of depression. *Can Med Assoc J.* **161**: 37–40.

54 Department of Health (2003) *Fast-Forwarding Primary Care Mental Health: graduate primary care mental health workers – best practice guidelines.* HMSO, London.

55 Department of Health (2002) *Fast-Forwarding Primary Care Mental Health – 'gateway' workers.* HMSO, London.

Postscript

We hope you have enjoyed reading this book. Clinical practice guidelines can improve the health of people with mental health problems, if they are rigorously developed, appropriately used and energetically implemented. We will have achieved our aim if you are now familiar with this process, and have taken away ideas for how you might use guidelines in your own practice.

We would particularly like to thank the chapter authors, who have pulled off that rare trick of covering this wide range of material while being both readable and authoritative. We have been honoured to collaborate with such eminent names in the field of guidelines development and use.

So what does the future hold for mental health clinical practice guidelines in the UK? As Professor Sir Michael Rawlins points out in his foreword, the UK NHS probably has the largest guideline development programme of any healthcare system in the world. However, the test for mental health, as with all other areas covered by guidelines, will be whether people's health improves as a result. NICE and SIGN have clearly demonstrated here that they have rigorous guideline development processes, yet the NCCMH has elucidated the problems for clinical practice guidelines in the mental health field. Guidelines will need to be credible with mental health clinicians and service users and carers alike. Probably the biggest challenge will be in their implementation on the ground. Many pointers from the evidence on 'what works' are provided here, but there is still a lot of research needed on how best to implement clinical practice guidelines. With the exception of depression guidelines in primary care, there is very little research on guidelines implementation in mental health. In our view, 'implementation research' in the mental health field deserves to be a research priority.

Paula Whitty
Martin Eccles
March 2004

Completed NICE mental health technology appraisals and guidelines: summaries as available from the NICE website*

Technology appraisals

Guidance on the use of newer (atypical) antipsychotic drugs for the treatment of schizophrenia[1]

(Excerpt from www.nice.org.uk/pdf/43_Antipsychotics_summary.pdf)

1 Guidance

1.1 The choice of antipsychotic drug should be made jointly by the individual and the clinician responsible for treatment based on an informed discussion of the relative benefits of the drugs and their side-effect profiles. The individual's advocate or carer should be consulted where appropriate.

1.2 It is recommended that the oral atypical antipsychotic drugs amisulpride, olanzapine, quetiapine, risperidone and zotepine are considered in the choice of first-line treatments for individuals with newly diagnosed schizophrenia.

1.3 The oral atypical antipsychotic drugs listed in Section 3.3 should be considered as treatment options for individuals currently receiving typical antipsychotic drugs who, despite adequate symptom control, are experiencing unacceptable side-effects, and for those in relapse who have previously experienced unsatisfactory management or unacceptable side-effects with typical antipsychotic drugs. The decision as to what are unacceptable side-effects should be taken following discussion between the patient and the clinician responsible for treatment.

---

* *Note*: The excerpts provided here are summaries only. The full documents are available on the NICE website at www.nice.org.uk or by telephoning (44) (0) 870 1555 455. The websites provided with the summaries refer to the documents that the excerpts were obtained from; the references provided at the end of the appendix refer to the full documents.

1.4 It is not recommended that, in routine clinical practice, individuals change to one of the oral atypical antipsychotic drugs if they are currently achieving good control of their condition without unacceptable side-effects with typical antipsychotic drugs.

1.5 In individuals with evidence of treatment-resistant schizophrenia (TRS), clozapine should be introduced at the earliest opportunity. TRS is suggested by a lack of satisfactory clinical improvement despite the sequential use of the recommended doses for 6 to 8 weeks of at least two antipsychotics, at least one of which should be an atypical.

1.6 A risk assessment should be performed by the clinician responsible for treatment and the multidisciplinary team regarding concordance with medication, and depot preparations should be prescribed when appropriate.

1.7 Where more than one atypical antipsychotic drug is considered appropriate, the drug with the lowest purchase cost (taking into account daily required dose and product price per dose) should be prescribed.

1.8 When full discussion between the clinician responsible for treatment and the individual concerned is not possible, in particular in the management of an acute schizophrenic episode, the oral atypical drugs should be considered as the treatment options of choice because of the lower potential risk of extrapyramidal symptoms (EPS). In these circumstances, the individual's carer or advocate should be consulted where possible and appropriate. Although there are limitations with advanced directives regarding the choice of treatment for individuals with schizophrenia, it is recommended that they are developed and documented in individuals' care programmes whenever possible.

1.9 Antipsychotic therapy should be initiated as part of a comprehensive package of care that addresses the individual's clinical, emotional and social needs. The clinician responsible for treatment and key worker should monitor both therapeutic progress and tolerability of the drug on an ongoing basis. Monitoring is particularly important when individuals have just changed from one antipsychotic to another.

1.10 Atypical and typical antipsychotic drugs should not be prescribed concurrently except for short periods to cover changeover of medication.

Guidance on the use of computerised cognitive behavioural therapy for anxiety and depression[2]

(Excerpt from www.nice.org.uk/pdf/51_CCBT_A4_summary.pdf)

1 Guidance

1.1 Current research suggests that the delivery of cognitive behavioural therapy via a computer interface (CCBT) may be of value in the management of anxiety and depressive disorders. This evidence is, however, an insufficient basis on which to recommend the general introduction of this technology into the NHS.

1.2 To establish the contribution and place of CCBT in the management of anxiety and depressive disorders, including its role within 'stepped care' approaches, the NHS should consider supporting an independent programme of research into CCBT, including carefully monitored pilot implementation projects. The research should include investigations into user preferences, suitability, needs and educational/cultural characteristics.

Guidance on the use of donepezil, rivastigmine and galantamine for Alzheimer's disease[3]

(Excerpt from www.nice.org.uk/pdf/ALZHEIMER_full_guidance.pdf)

1 Guidance

1.1 The three drugs donepezil, rivastigmine and galantamine should be made available in the NHS as one component of the management of those people with mild and moderate Alzheimer's disease (AD) whose mini mental state examination (MMSE) score is above 12 points (*see* paragraph 2.6 and 4.3) under the following conditions:

1.1.1 Diagnosis that the form of dementia is AD must be made in a specialist clinic according to standard diagnostic criteria.

1.1.2 Assessment in a specialist clinic, including tests of cognitive, global and behavioural functioning and of activities of daily living, should be made before the drug is prescribed.

1.1.3 Clinicians should also exercise judgement about the likelihood of compliance; in general, a carer or care-worker who is in sufficient contact with the patient to ensure compliance should be a minimum requirement.

1.1.4 Only specialists (including old age psychiatrists, neurologists, and care of the elderly physicians) should initiate treatment. Carers' views of the patient's condition at base-line and follow-up should be sought. If general practitioners are to take over prescribing, it is recommended that they should do so under an agreed shared-care protocol with clear treatment end points.

1.1.5 A further assessment should be made, usually 2 to 4 months after reaching maintenance dose of the drug. Following this assessment the drug should be continued only where there has been an improvement or no deterioration in MMSE score, together with evidence of global improvement on the basis of behavioural and/or functional assessment.

1.1.6 Patients who continue on the drug should be reviewed by MMSE score and global, functional and behavioural assessment every 6 months. The drug should normally only be continued while their MMSE score remains above 12 points, and their global, functional and behavioural condition remains at a level where the drug is considered to be having a worthwhile effect. When the MMSE score falls below 12 points, patients should not normally be prescribed any of these three drugs. Any review involving MMSE assessment should be undertaken by an appropriate specialist team, unless there are locally-agreed protocols for shared care.

1.2 The benefits of these three drugs for patients with other forms of dementia (e.g. Dementia with Lewy Bodies) has not been assessed in this guidance.

Guidance on the use of methylphenidate (Ritalin, Equasym) for attention deficit/hyperactivity disorder (ADHD) in childhood[4]

(Excerpt from www.nice.org.uk/article.asp?a=11667)

1 Guidance

1.1 Methylphenidate is recommended for use as part of a comprehensive treatment programme for children with a diagnosis of severe attention deficit/hyperactivity disorder (ADHD). 'Severe ADHD' is broadly similar to a diagnosis of hyperkinetic disorder (HKD), although in some cases treatment may be appropriate for children and adolescents who do not fit the diagnostic criteria for HKD but are experiencing severe problems due to inattention or hyperactivity/impulsiveness.

1.2 Methylphenidate is not currently licensed for children under the age of six or for children with marked anxiety, agitation or tension; symptoms or family history of tics or Tourette's syndrome; hyperthyroidism; severe angina or cardiac arrhythmia; glaucoma; or thyrotoxicosis. Caution is required in the prescribing of methylphenidate for children and young people with epilepsy, psychotic disorders, or a history of drug or alcohol dependence.

1.3 Diagnosis should be based on a timely, comprehensive assessment conducted by a child/adolescent psychiatrist or a paediatrician with expertise in ADHD. It should also involve children, parents and carers and the child's school, and take into account cultural factors in the child's environment. Multidisciplinary assessment, which may include educational or clinical psychologists and social workers, is advisable for children who present with indications of significant comorbidity.

1.4 Treatment with methylphenidate should only be initiated by child and adolescent psychiatrists or paediatricians with expertise in ADHD, but continued prescribing and monitoring may be performed by general practitioners, under shared care arrangements with specialists.

1.5 Careful titration is required to determine the optimal dose level and timing. The drug should be discontinued if improvement of symptoms is not observed after appropriate dose adjustment.

1.6 A comprehensive treatment programme should involve advice and support to parents and teachers, and could, but does not need to, include specific psychological treatment (such as behavioural therapy). While this wider service is desirable, any shortfall in its provision should not be used as a reason for delaying the appropriate use of medication.

1.7 Children on methylphenidate therapy should receive regular monitoring. When improvement has occurred and the child's condition is stable, treatment can be discontinued at intervals, under careful specialist supervision, in order to assess both the child's progress and the need for continuation of therapy.

1.8 This guidance relates only to children and adolescents with ADHD.

Guidance on the use of electroconvulsive therapy[5]

(Excerpt from www.nice.org.uk/pdf/59ecta4summary.pdf)

1.1 It is recommended that electroconvulsive therapy (ECT) is used only to achieve rapid and short-term improvement of severe symptoms after an adequate trial of other treatment options has proven ineffective and/or when the condition is considered to be potentially life-threatening, in individuals with:

• severe depressive illness
• catatonia
• a prolonged or severe manic episode.

1.2 The decision as to whether ECT is clinically indicated should be based on a documented assessment of the risks and potential benefits to the individual, including: the risks associated with the anaesthetic; current comorbidities; anticipated adverse events, particularly cognitive impairment; and the risks of not having treatment.

1.3 The risks associated with ECT may be enhanced during pregnancy, in older people, and in children and young people, and therefore clinicians should exercise particular caution when considering ECT treatment in these groups.

1.4 Valid consent should be obtained in all cases where the individual has the ability to grant or refuse consent. The decision to use ECT should be made jointly by the individual and the clinician(s) responsible for treatment, on the basis of an informed discussion. This discussion should be enabled by the provision of full and appropriate information about the general risks associated with ECT (*see* Section 1.9) and about the risks and potential benefits specific to that individual. Consent should be obtained without pressure or coercion, which may occur as a result of the circumstances and clinical setting, and the individual should be reminded of their right to withdraw consent at any point. There should be strict adherence to recognised guidelines about consent and the involvement of patient advocates and/or carers to facilitate informed discussion is strongly encouraged.

1.5 In all situations where informed discussion and consent is not possible, advance directives should be taken fully into account and the individual's advocate and/or carer should be consulted.

1.6 Clinical status should be assessed following each ECT session and treatment should be stopped when a response has been achieved, or sooner if there is evidence of adverse effects. Cognitive function should be monitored on an ongoing basis, and at a minimum at the end of each course of treatment.

1.7 It is recommended that a repeat course of ECT should be considered under the circumstances indicated in 1.1 only for individuals who have severe depressive illness, catatonia or mania and who have previously responded well to ECT. In patients who are experiencing an acute episode but have not previously responded, a repeat trial of ECT should be undertaken only after all other options have been considered and following discussion of the risks and benefits with the individual and/or where appropriate their carer/advocate.

1.8 As the longer-term benefits and risks of ECT have not been clearly established, it is not recommended as a maintenance therapy in depressive illness.

1.9 The current state of the evidence does not allow the general use of ECT in the management of schizophrenia to be recommended.

1.10 National information leaflets should be developed through consultation with appropriate professional and user organisations to enable individuals and their carers/advocates to make an informed decision regarding the appropriateness of ECT for their circumstances. The leaflets should be evidence based, include information about the risks of ECT and availability of alternative treatments, and be produced in formats and languages that make them accessible to a wide range of service users.

NEW DRUGS FOR BIPOLAR DISORDERS

Olanzapine and valproate sodium in the treatment of acute mania associated with bipolar I disorder[6]

(Excerpt from www.nice.org.uk/pdf/66_bipolardisorder_A4summary.pdf)

1 Guidance

1.1 Olanzapine and valproate semisodium, within their licensed indications, are recommended as options for control of the acute symptoms associated with the manic phase of bipolar I disorder.

1.2 Of the drugs available for the treatment of acute mania, the choice of which to prescribe should be made jointly by the individual and the clinician(s) responsible for treatment. The choice should be based on an informed discussion of the relative benefits and side-effect profiles of each drug, and should take into account the needs of the individual and the particular clinical situation.

1.3 In all situations where informed discussion is not possible advance directives should be taken fully into account and the individual's advocate and/or carer should be consulted when appropriate.

1.4 At the date of issue of this guidance, within the classes of agents referred to the Institute by the Department of Health and the Welsh Assembly Government, only olanzapine and valproate semisodium held a marketing authorisation for the treatment of acute mania in bipolar I disorder.

Guidelines

Schizophrenia: core interventions in the treatment and management of schizophrenia in primary and secondary care[7]

(Excerpts from www.nice.org.uk/pdf/schizophreniascope.pdf; www.nice.org.uk/pdf/media_briefing_FINAL.pdf; www.nice.org.uk/Docref.asp?d=42460)*

---

* *Note*: There is no summary version available for this guideline, therefore excerpts from the scope for the guideline, press briefing released at the time of guideline publication, and from the introduction to the full guideline, are provided here.

2 Notes on the scope of the guidance

2.1 This guideline is relevant to adults (>18 years) with a diagnosis of schizophrenia with the onset before 60 years of age, and for all healthcare professionals involved in the help, treatment and care of people with schizophrenia and their carers. These include:

• adults with a diagnosis of schizophrenia and their families/carers
• professional groups who share in the treatment and care for people with a diagnosis of schizophrenia, including psychiatrists, clinical psychologists, mental health nurses, community psychiatric nurses, social workers, practice nurses, occupational therapists, pharmacists and GPs
• professionals in other health and non-health sectors who may have direct contact with or be involved in the provision of health and other public services for those diagnosed with schizophrenia. These may include A&E staff, paramedical staff, prison doctors, the police and persons who work in the criminal justice and education sectors
• those with responsibility for planning services for people with a diagnosis of schizophrenia, and their carers, including directors of public health, NHS trust managers and managers in primary care trusts.

2.2 The guidance does not specifically address the treatment and management of people with:

• very-early onset (childhood-onset) schizophrenia
• very-late onset (age of onset at 60 years of age or greater) schizophrenia
• schizophrenia with co-existing learning difficulties
• schizophrenia with co-existing substance misuse
• schizophrenia with co-existing significant physical or sensory difficulties
• schizophrenics who are homeless.

2.3 Although this guideline briefly addresses the issue of diagnosis, it has not made evidence-based recommendations nor has it referred to evidence regarding diagnosis, primary prevention or assessment.

[This] guideline *Schizophrenia: core interventions in the treatment and management of schizophrenia in primary and secondary care*, outlines best practice for health professionals caring for individuals with schizophrenia in a range of areas, including:

• care across all stages (for example, the importance of working in partnership with service users and carers, and offering treatment in an atmosphere of hope and optimism)
• initiation of treatment (for example, the development of early intervention services to provide appropriate care for people with suspected or newly diagnosed schizophrenia)

- treatment of acute episodes (for example, the use of antipsychotic drugs as part of a comprehensive package of care that addresses the individual's clinical, emotional and social needs)
- promoting recovery (for example, the use of psychological interventions such as cognitive behavioural therapy to prevent relapse and reduce symptoms)
- rapid tranquillisation (for example, minimising factors that might increase need for rapid tranquillisation and outlining the principles health professionals should follow).

For the purposes of this guideline, the treatment and management of schizophrenia has been divided into three phases:

- initiation of treatment at the first episode
- acute phase
- promoting recovery.

The guideline makes good practice points and recommendations for psychological, pharmacological and service-level interventions in the three phases of care in both primary care and secondary mental health services. Drugs considered in this guideline are restricted to those licensed for use in the UK prior to May 2002, and the psychological treatments dealt with here are for use in addition to antipsychotic medication.

Eating disorders: core interventions in the treatment and management of anorexia nervosa, bulimia nervosa and related eating disorders[8]

(Excerpt from www.nice.org.uk/pdf/cg009quickrefguide.pdf)

Key priorities for implementation
The following recommendations have been identified as key priorities for implementation.

Anorexia nervosa
- Most people with anorexia nervosa should be managed on an outpatient basis with psychological treatment provided by a service that is competent in giving that treatment and assessing the physical risk of people with eating disorders.
- People with anorexia nervosa requiring inpatient treatment should be admitted to a setting that can provide the skilled implementation of refeeding with careful physical monitoring (particularly in the first few days of refeeding) in combination with psychosocial interventions.
- Family interventions that directly address the eating disorder should be offered to children and adolescents with anorexia nervosa.

Bulimia nervosa
- As a possible first step, patients with bulimia nervosa should be encouraged to follow an evidence-based self-help programme.
- As an alternative or additional first step to using an evidence-based self-help programme, adults with bulimia nervosa may be offered a trial of an antidepressant drug.
- Cognitive behaviour therapy for bulimia nervosa (CBT-BN), a specifically adapted form of CBT, should be offered to adults with bulimia nervosa. The course of treatment should be for 16 to 20 sessions over 4 to 5 months.
- Adolescents with bulimia nervosa may be treated with CBT-BN, adapted as needed to suit their age, circumstances and level of development, and including the family as appropriate.

Atypical eating disorders
- In the absence of evidence to guide the management of atypical eating disorders (eating disorders not otherwise specified) other than binge eating disorder, it is recommended that the clinician considers following the guidance on the treatment of the eating problem that most closely resembles the individual patient's eating disorder.
- Cognitive behaviour therapy for binge eating disorder (CBT-BED), a specifically adapted form of CBT, should be offered to adults with binge eating disorder.

For all eating disorders
- Family members including siblings should normally be included in the treatment of children and adolescents with eating disorders. Interventions may include sharing of information, advice on behavioural management and facilitating communication.

References

1   National Institute for Clinical Excellence (2002) *Guidance on the use of newer (atypical) antipsychotic drugs for the treatment of schizophrenia.* NICE, London. www.nice.org/uk/Docref.asp?d=32922

2   National Institute for Clinical Excellence (2002) *Guidance on the use of computerised cognitive behavioural therapy for anxiety and depression.* NICE, London. www.nice.org.uk/Docref.asp?d=38248

3   National Institute for Clinical Excellence (2001) *Guidance on the use of donepezil, rivastigmine and galantamine for Alzheimer's disease.* NICE, London. www.nice.org.uk/Docref.asp?d=14412

4   National Institute for Clinical Excellence (2000) *Guidance on the use of methylphenidate (Ritalin, Equasym) for attention deficit/hyperactivity disorder (ADHD) in childhood.* NICE, London. www.nice.org.uk/Docref.asp?d=11653

5 National Institute for Clinical Excellence (2003) *Guidance on the use of electroconvulsive therapy.* NICE, London. www.nice.org.uk/Docref.asp?d=68306

6 National Institute for Clinical Excellence (2003) *Olanzapine and valproate sodium in the treatment of acute mania associated with bipolar I disorder.* NICE, London. www.nice.org.uk/Docref.asp?d=86783

7 National Institute for Clinical Excellence (2002) *Schizophrenia: core interventions in the treatment and management of schizophrenia in primary and secondary care.* NICE, London. www.nice.org.uk/Docref.asp?d=42460

8 National Institute for Clinical Excellence (2004) *Eating disorders: core interventions in the treatment and management of anorexia nervosa, bulimia nervosa and related eating disorders.* NICE, London. www.nice.org.uk/Docref.asp?d=101245

Index